OBSTETRICS AND GYNECOLOGY ADVANCES

PREECLAMPSIA

RISK FACTORS, PATHOGENESIS AND POTENTIAL TREATMENTS

OBSTETRICS AND GYNECOLOGY ADVANCES

Additional books and e-books in this series can be found on Nova's website under the Series tab.

OBSTETRICS AND GYNECOLOGY ADVANCES

PREECLAMPSIA

RISK FACTORS, PATHOGENESIS AND POTENTIAL TREATMENTS

TORSTEN NACHT
EDITOR

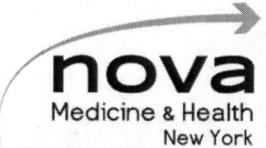

Copyright © 2020 by Nova Science Publishers, Inc.

All rights reserved. No part of this book may be reproduced, stored in a retrieval system or transmitted in any form or by any means: electronic, electrostatic, magnetic, tape, mechanical photocopying, recording or otherwise without the written permission of the Publisher.

We have partnered with Copyright Clearance Center to make it easy for you to obtain permissions to reuse content from this publication. Simply navigate to this publication's page on Nova's website and locate the "Get Permission" button below the title description. This button is linked directly to the title's permission page on copyright.com. Alternatively, you can visit copyright.com and search by title, ISBN, or ISSN.

For further questions about using the service on copyright.com, please contact:
Copyright Clearance Center
Phone: +1-(978) 750-8400   Fax: +1-(978) 750-4470   E-mail: info@copyright.com.

NOTICE TO THE READER

The Publisher has taken reasonable care in the preparation of this book, but makes no expressed or implied warranty of any kind and assumes no responsibility for any errors or omissions. No liability is assumed for incidental or consequential damages in connection with or arising out of information contained in this book. The Publisher shall not be liable for any special, consequential, or exemplary damages resulting, in whole or in part, from the readers' use of, or reliance upon, this material. Any parts of this book based on government reports are so indicated and copyright is claimed for those parts to the extent applicable to compilations of such works.

Independent verification should be sought for any data, advice or recommendations contained in this book. In addition, no responsibility is assumed by the Publisher for any injury and/or damage to persons or property arising from any methods, products, instructions, ideas or otherwise contained in this publication.

This publication is designed to provide accurate and authoritative information with regard to the subject matter covered herein. It is sold with the clear understanding that the Publisher is not engaged in rendering legal or any other professional services. If legal or any other expert assistance is required, the services of a competent person should be sought. FROM A DECLARATION OF PARTICIPANTS JOINTLY ADOPTED BY A COMMITTEE OF THE AMERICAN BAR ASSOCIATION AND A COMMITTEE OF PUBLISHERS.

Additional color graphics may be available in the e-book version of this book.

Library of Congress Cataloging-in-Publication Data

ISBN: 978-1-53617-116-7

Published by Nova Science Publishers, Inc. † New York

CONTENTS

Preface		vii
Chapter 1	Evaluation of Early Markers of Preeclampsia *Svetlana Dubrovina, Vitaliy Gimbut and Ulduz Mutsalkhanova*	1
Chapter 2	Preeclampsia Pathogenesis *Nese Colcimen*	19
Chapter 3	Pre-Eclampsia: Prediction, Prevention and Treatment *I. V. Lakhno*	37
Chapter 4	Pre-eclampsia Management Problems Today *Alena I. Baranouskaya*	53
Bibliography		79
Related Nova Publications		165
Index		179

PREFACE

Preeclampsia: Risk Factors, Pathogenesis and Potential Treatments investigates the clinical, anamnestic, and biochemical predictors of preeclampsia. As such, a prognostic model based on the co-use of the studied predictors has been developed for the early prediction of late-onset moderate preeclampsia.

The authors summarize some theories suggested to explain the pathogenesis of preeclampsia. The pathogenesis of preeclampsia has not yet been fully clarified and it remains a disease of theories. Furthermore, as it is a human-specific disease, the lack of one-on-one animal modeling and many other factors contribute to poor understanding of the disease pathophysiology.

Additionally, this collection explores the possibilities of the maternal and fetal heart rate variability usage at all stages of management among pre-eclamptic women in a three-stage system.

The concluding review includes sources of literature on the pathogenesis, management and long-term consequences of pre-eclampsia.

Chapter 1 - *Objective*. The aim of the study was to investigate the clinical, anamnestic, and biochemical predictors of preeclampsia.

Subjects and methods. Clinical, anamnestic, and biochemical examinations were performed in the first trimester in pregnant women, who later (after delivery) formed two groups: with late-onset moderate preeclampsia and without preeclampsia.

Results. Significant clinical markers for late-onset preeclampsia showed increases in body mass index and mean blood pressure at 11-13 weeks of gestation. Additionally, the pregnant women with preeclampsia were found to have significantly higher serum levels of retinol-binding protein 4, disintegrin, and metalloproteinase 12. The anamnestic predictors of preeclampsia were ascertained to be a history of hypertension, chronic pyelonephritis, and preeclampsia in previous pregnancies.

Conclusion. A prognostic model based on the co-use of the studied predictors has been developed for the early prediction of late-onset moderate preeclampsia.

Chapter 2 - Preeclampsia is usually defined as new-onset hypertension and proteinuria diagnosed at 20th gestational week or after. Preeclampsia is one of the leading causes of maternal and infant mortality worldwide. It is important to clarify its pathogenesis for its treatment and prevention. This chapter summarized some theories suggested to explain the pathogenesis of preeclampsia. The pathogenesis of preeclampsia has not yet been fully clarified and it remains a disease of theories. Furthermore, as it is a human-specific disease, the lack of one-on-one animal modeling and many other factors contribute to poor understanding of the disease pathophysiology. For this reason, continuous efforts have been made and new theories have been put forth to explain the disease pathophysiology. New data have revealed the unknowns and guide our understanding about the mechanism of the multifactorial pathogenesis of the disease. Our hope is that the accumulation of knowledge on the subject will clarify the pathogenesis of the disease and make us reach a definitive conclusion in the treatment and prevention of the disease in the near future.

Chapter 3 - The chapter covers the possibilities of the maternal and fetal heart rate variability usage at all stages of management among pre-eclamptic women in a three-stage system.

It has been shown that pre-eclampsia is featured by sympathetic overactivity, vascular spasm, and reduced cardiac output influenced by increased intra-abdominal pressure. The deterioration of uteroplacental circulation was found to decrease the penetration of maternal respiratory sinus arrhythmia through the placental barrier among women with a hypokinetic type of central maternal hemodynamics. These events are captured in the development of maternal multiple organ failure and fetal distress.

The usage of variables of autonomic balance has improved the predictive value of traditional screening of pre-eclampsia by 4.5 times. The application of combined pharmaceutical prophylactics has contributed to the reduction of pre-eclampsia by 8.25 times. The additional screening at 26–28 weeks of pregnancy included maternal heart rate variability parameters which made the selection of contingent for preterm delivery more reasonable.

Chapter 4 - This review includes sources of literature with a purpose of the systematization of modern information on pathogenesis, management and the long-term consequences of pre-eclampsia. There is scientific evidence of the role of soluble Fms-like tyrosine kinase-1and angiogenic growth factors in the pathogenesis of preeclampsia. However, modern science does not exactly know the etiology of preeclampsia. Therefore, the only way of terminating preeclampsia is giving a childbirth. Successful management of preeclampsia involves coherent, correct steps. In a patient with arterial hypertension, it is necessary to conduct a differential diagnosis, assess the severity of preeclampsia and confirm the condition of the fetus. Criteria for the diagnosis of preeclampsia are known, but problems with the treatment of this pathology still remains. Delivery is necessary for women with severe or progressive preeclampsia. In all countries, it is recommended to use magnesium sulphate for the prevention and treatment of eclampsia and to use corticosteroids for prevention neonatal complications in case of premature pregnancy. The long-term consequences of preeclampsia are cardiovascular diseases and the resulting death.

In: Preeclampsia
Editor: Torsten Nacht

ISBN: 978-1-53617-116-7
© 2020 Nova Science Publishers, Inc.

Chapter 1

EVALUATION OF EARLY MARKERS OF PREECLAMPSIA

Svetlana Dubrovina[1,*]*, PhD, Vitaliy Gimbut*[1]*, PhD and Ulduz Mutsalkhanova*[1]*, PhD*
[1]Rostov Scientific Institute of Obstetrics and Pediatrics,
Rostov State Medical University, Rostov-on-Don, Russia

ABSTRACT

Objective. The aim of the study was to investigate the clinical, anamnestic, and biochemical predictors of preeclampsia.

Subjects and methods. Clinical, anamnestic, and biochemical examinations were performed in the first trimester in pregnant women, who later (after delivery) formed two groups: with late-onset moderate preeclampsia and without preeclampsia.

Results. Significant clinical markers for late-onset preeclampsia showed increases in body mass index and mean blood pressure at 11-13 weeks of gestation. Additionally, the pregnant women with preeclampsia were found to have significantly higher serum levels of retinol-binding protein 4, disintegrin, and metalloproteinase 12. The anamnestic

---

[*] E-mail: s.dubrovina@gmail.com.

predictors of preeclampsia were ascertained to be a history of hypertension, chronic pyelonephritis, and preeclampsia in previous pregnancies.

Conclusion. A prognostic model based on the co-use of the studied predictors has been developed for the early prediction of late-onset moderate preeclampsia.

Keywords: pregnancy, preeclampsia, early predictors

INTRODUCTION

Despite the achievements of medical science, preeclampsia remains one of the main causes of maternal and infant morbidity and mortality in contemporary obstetrics.

Preeclampsia (PE) affects about 2% of pregnancies and remains a major cause of maternal and perinatal morbidity and mortality [1, 2]. However, currently we can observe a certain progress in the research of origin mechanisms of this threatening complication of gestation, and this is connected with a change in the understanding of preeclampsia's initial forming period [3].

PE can be classified into early and late onset, and it is widely accepted that these subtypes of PE are different forms of the disease. Early-onset PE, regarding delivery before 34 weeks' gestation, is commonly associated with intrauterine growth retardation (IUGR), abnormal uterine and umbilical artery Doppler waveforms, and adverse maternal and neonatal outcomes. To the contrary, late-onset PE, with delivery at a period of 34 weeks or after, is mostly associated with mild maternal disease and a low rate of fetal involvement. The perinatal outcomes of late-onset PE are usually favorable [4]. The concept of early or late beginnings reflects differences in the pathophysiology of preeclampsia. Numerous works have demonstrated differences in the causes of the disease origins: early preeclampsia is preconditioned by placentation abnormalities, and late PE is connected, as a rule, with maternal factors [5, 6]. Early preeclampsia is witnessed more rarely but has more negative consequences for mother and fetus [7].

Nevertheless, considerable achievements in the study of pathogeneses of the given complication of gestation haven't decreased the frequency of its occurrence so far. In practical terms there is observed an absence of a systematic approach in terms of prenatal care tactics towards women under the threat of preeclampsia, together with the very limited use of preeclampsia markers, discovered in the run of scientific studies. Moreover, many questions concerning the etiopathogenetic factors of preeclampsia still remain in dispute. Thus, the search for early predictors for preeclampsia prognosis, being efficient and affordable, remains a priority task for modern obstetrics.

The aim of the current study is to define clinical-anamnestic and biochemical predictors of preeclampsia, with the purpose of modernizing its early prognosis and prevention methods.

MÉTHODES

Participants

In order to solve the tasks in hand on the basis of perspective analysis of clinical data, 25 women with preeclampsia, belonging to the first (main) clinical group, were selected out of the total number of women ($n = 645$), who were being observed throughout the whole gestation period. The patients taking part in the study suffered from moderately severe preeclampsia, which appeared after 34 weeks of pregnancy (late preeclampsia). The second (control) group included 63 patients without preeclampsia, were chosen using the random numbers method.

All the pregnant women were subjected to a complex set of clinical, anamnestic, and instrumental tests in the dynamics of gestation. Screening blood sampling was carried out within the period of 11 - 13 weeks of pregnancy. The women of the chosen groups underwent enzyme immunoassay to define biochemical markers in their blood serum:

placental protein A (PAPP-A), associated with pregnancy, disintegrin and metalloproteinase 12 (ADAM12), retinol-connecting protein 4 (RBP4), ®-subunit human chorionic gonadotropin (®-HCG), and cystatin C. The choice of the present array of clinical and biochemical parameters was made on the basis of literature data analysis [8-14].

The level of ADAM12 was established by test-systems Cloud-CloneCorp (USA), cystatin C by test-systems BioVendor (Czech Republic), RBP4 by test-systems AssayPro (USA), ®-HCG and PAPP-A by test-systems DELFIA PerkinElmer (Finland).

Statistic processing of the data was carried out with the use of the programs Statistica, version 12.5, Excel 2010, and SPSS 24.002. Within the compared groups median values, we assessed at 25% and 75% percentage calculation (1 - 3 quartile) for getting quantitative indicators. While comparing inter-group difference, non-parametric criteria for the independent samples by Craskal-Wallis was used. Fisher's criteria (φ) was used to compare the occurrence frequency of the given indices of the two picks. Additionally, a non-parametric correlation analysis with the application of Spearmen criteria, together with the "Solution trees" method, was used in order to attribute certain objects to one of the preliminarily familiar classes.

Results and Discussion

The following facts have been discovered in the process of analyzing clinical-anamnestic data. When comparing height-weight indices of the chosen groups it was found that body mass index (BMI) of the patients with preeclampsia within the period of 11 - 13 weeks of pregnancy is statistically much higher than that of patients from the control group. BMI in the early periods of gestation for the patients with preeclampsia was 29kg\m2, while for the patients from the control group it was 25kg\m2 ($p = 0.0001$). A population-based study of 159,072 singleton births in the USA revealed that not only obese women (pre-pregnancy body mass index [BMI] $\geq$ 30.0), but also overweight women (pre-pregnancy BMI = 25.0 –

29.9) were at a significantly higher risk for preeclampsia (odds ratio 2.0 and 3.3, respectively) than women with a pre-pregnancy BMI of less than 20.0 [15]. Our study confirmed the role of BMI as an independent factor of preeclampsia development.

Analysis of anamnestic data revealed that for most of the women participating in the research this was a second pregnancy, both in the control group and in the group of women with preeclampsia (49 (78%) and 20 (80%); p = 0,. 78). The number of women with a first pregnancy in the observed groups was also similar (14 (22%) and 5 (20%); p = 0.688). It's known that preeclampsia in anamnesis is a prognostic factor for preeclampsia development in the case of real pregnancy. Within the research 5 (20%) of the pregnant women from the main group had preeclampsia in anamnesis, while in the control group there were 2 women with such anamnesis (3%) (p = 0.009). For 4 (16%) of the patients with preeclampsia, anamnestic data contained information about chronic endometritis, which is positively more frequent than in the control group – 2 (4%) (p = 0.0001). Abortion in anamnesis was observed for 7 (28%) of patients in the main group, and 21 (33%) of patients in the control group (p > 0.05). Analysis of occurrence of extra-genital pathology revealed considerable differences for chronic pyelonephritis (6 (24%) and 8 (13%); p = 0.010), and arterial hypertension in anamnesis (10 (40%) and 8 (13%); p = 0.0001). According to the literature data [5, 16], there is a higher risk of preeclampsia during pregnancy in patients with arterial hypertension in anamnesis. The results of the given study confirm the data of S. Iacobelli and co-authors, which demonstrated that burdened somatic anamnesis, including both arterial hypertension and kidney pathology, is a risk factor for preeclampsia development [17].

The next comparison parameter was medium arterial pressure (MAP), which was calculated with the help of the formula: (2 figures of diastolic arterial pressure) + (figures of systolic arterial pressure))/3. Comparative analysis of MAP revealed much higher figures for the pregnant women with preeclampsia. Additionally, a strong correlation between a group of signs (MAP, BMI), and subgroups with preeclampsia and nominally healthy people, was revealed (table 1).

Table 1. Estimation criteria of power of correlation between risk factors (MAP, BMI) and the outcome for the chosen clinical groups

Criteria	Criteria value	Correlation power*
Criteria of φ (Fisher)	0.543	Relatively Strong
Coefficient of contingency of Pearson (C)	0.477	Relatively strong
Normalized value of Pearson coefficient (C')	0.675	Strong

*Interpretation of the received indices of statistical criteria according to the recommendations of Rea & Parker.

The figures for MAP were considerably higher for the patients with preeclampsia (84 [75; 93]mm Hg) in comparison with patients from the control group (78 [73; 83]mm Hg, p = 0.0082). According to the data, provided by D. Gallo with his co-authors [2], based on observation of 17,383 pregnant women, MAP figures also had high prognostic efficiency concerning preeclampsia.

Our study revealed higher occurrence of threatened abortion and premature delivery for women with preeclampsia in comparison with the patients of the control group (12 (48%) and 13 (21%); $p = 0.010$), and also an increase in frequency of caesarean section for pregnant patients with preeclampsia (14 (56%) versus 9 (14%), $p = 0.010$). Taking into account the professional literature, a threatened abortion in the first trimester is closely connected with the pathological progress of gestation, as the development of pregnancy initially takes place under unfavorable conditions and is accompanied by impaired trophoblast invasion [17].

Thus, analysis of clinical-anamnestic data allowed for the designation of a number of characteristics, statistically considerably differentiating patients from the chosen clinical groups, namely: presence of preeclampsia, chronic pyelonephritis and arterial hypertension, high indices for BMI in the beginning of pregnancy, MAP figures in the early stages of pregnancy, and complications in the progress of current pregnancy, such as threatened abortion and premature delivery. Analysis of the data allowed for the recommendation of the indicated factors, which predict development of late preeclampsia of medium severity, for further use. The advantage of the given screening is the absence of additional temporary and financial expenses for the examination, and the simplicity of its performance. With the combination of the offered parameters, doctors will be able to estimate the risk of preeclampsia development and make decisions about the necessity of applying additional predictors.

The next task of our work was to identify early biochemical correlators of preeclampsia. Currently, despite scientists' efforts, there aren't any biochemical markers that match the definition of the World Healthcare Organization for the selection of biomarkers, which either forecast or make a diagnosis for preeclampsia. We carried out an analysis of concentrations of PAPP-A, ADAM12, RBP4, ®-HCG and cystatin C in the venous blood of patients from the chosen groups as possible predictors of preeclampsia (table 2).

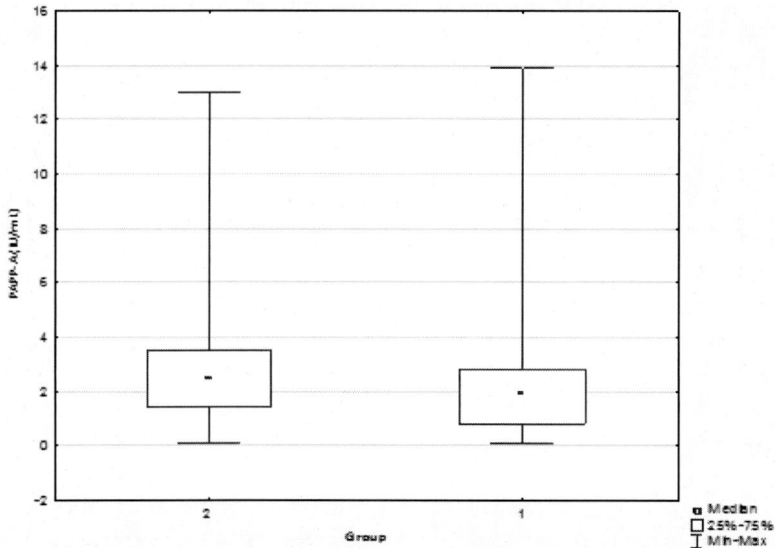

Figure 1. Pregnancy associated plasma protein-A (PAPP-A) levels in study groups.

One of the possible correlators of preeclampsia was PAPP-A, used as a biochemical marker for chromosome anomalies, especially in those with Down syndrome. It is measured during the second trimester of pregnancy. Additionally, low PAPP-A levels are associated with chromosomal anomalies in fetuses, and they can predict adverse pregnancy outcomes such as fetal growth restriction, spontaneous miscarriage, moderately and extremely premature births, PE, and stillbirths [8]. Comparative analysis of PAPP-A among pregnant women from those chosen for our study groups revealed an absence of substantial differences (1.92 [0.80; 2.82] IU/mL and 2.26 [1.14; 3.84] IU/mL; p = 0.269). The results correlate with the data of some authors [9] who deny the prognostic value of PAPP-A among patients with late preeclampsia.

Table 2. Biochemical indices for pregnant women from chosen groups

Biomarker, unit of measurement	Women groups		P
	I group (n = 25)	II group (n = 63)	
PAPP-A (IU/mL)	1.92 [0.80; 2.82]	2.26 [1.14; 3.84]	0.269
ADAM12 (ng/mL)	1,79 [0.93; 2.30]	0,84 [0.48; 1.29]	0.0001
Cystatin C (ng/mL)	524.26 [425.44; 576.33]	535.50 [484.62; 626.04]	0.160
RBP4 (ug/mL)	44.36 [34.95; 48.52]	32.53 [25.81; 36.29]	0.0003
ß-HCG (ng/ml)	38.98 [17.60; 46.50]	30.20 [21.60; 60.30]	0.544

Indication: p – level of meaningfulness of differences between groups, interquartile amplitude is noted in brackets.

The next biomarker of comparison is ADAM12, which participates in the breakdown of protein by binding insulin growth factor binding protein-3 [10]. This factor indirectly affects the interaction between the trophoblast and the maternal decidual cells and thus contributes to the proper mechanism of development of the chorionic vascular system and the placenta.

The level of ADAM12 (1.79 [0.93; 2.30]) for women with preeclampsia was considerably higher (p < 0,001), than in the control group (0.84 [0.48; 1.29]). The study by E. Matwejew and co-authors revealed increased levels of ADAM12 among women with preeclampsia in comparison with the control group [11]. The results of the given study confirmed the meaningfulness of ADAM12 as a possible early marker of development of late preeclampsia of medium severity.

RBP4, being one of adipokines, plays a crucial role in the development of resistance towards insulin, metabolism of lipids, atherosclerosis, and system inflammatory response.

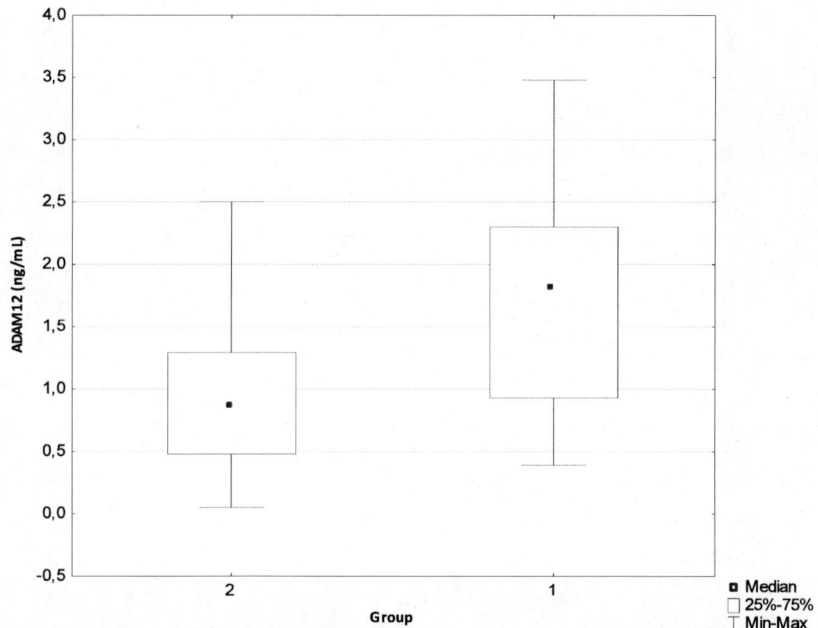

Figure 2. ADAM 12 levels in patient groups.

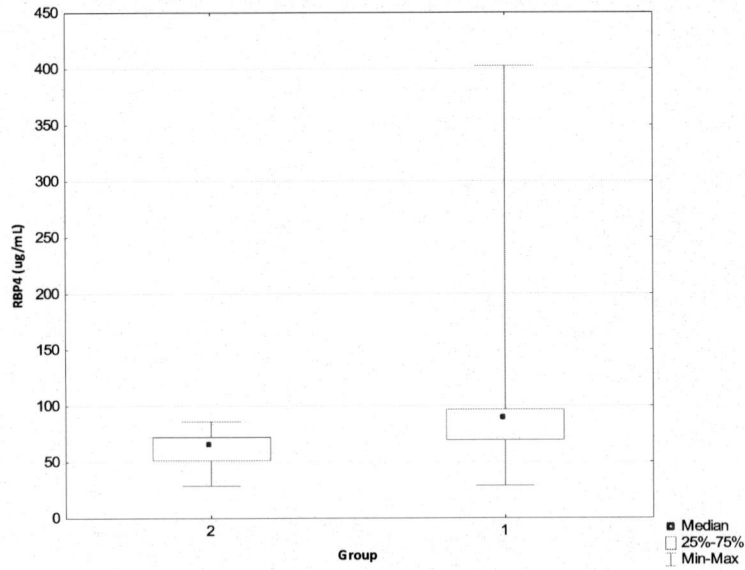

Figure 3. RBP4 Levels in study groups.

Identifying RBP4 in our work demonstrated that pregnant women with late preeclampsia of medium severity were characterized by higher levels of this parameter (44.36 [34.95; 48.52]ug/mL) in comparison with women from the control group (32.53 [25.81; 36.29]ug/mL).

According to the investigation by P. Mendola and co-authors [18], RBP4 concentrations at baseline and mid-pregnancy were associated with a 4- to 8-fold increase in preterm preeclampsia risk but were not associated with term preeclampsia. In another study [19] the role of RBP4 for early diagnosing of preeclampsia was also proven. PE patients had significantly higher serum RBP4 levels when compared to the corresponding levels of the control group. Serum levels of RBP4 showed positive significant correlation with diastolic blood pressures, extent of proteinuria, and patients' body weight measures. So, RBP4 was associated with the development and severity of PE.

According to another investigation [20], mean maternal RBP4 concentrations were not significantly different in PE (24.5mg/L) as compared to controls (22.3mg/L). Furthermore, RBP4 did not correlate to clinical and biochemical measures of pregnancy outcome, renal function, glucose and lipid metabolism, or inflammation. So, these results do not support a role of RBP4 in the pathogenesis of PE.

Some studies revealed that placental expression of cystatin C increases with preeclampsia [21], which leads to an increase of this marker level in blood plasma [22]. Our work demonstrated that the level of cystatin C in the blood of patients with preeclampsia didn't differ substantially from the levels of the control group (p = 0.160).

Similar results with an absence of statistical difference between patients of both groups (p = 0.544) were received for the level of ®-HCG. A large cohort study of IVF pregnancies [23] found an association between low HCG levels on day 12 after embryos transfer, and subsequent development of preeclampsia.

The results of this study are consistent with the literature in demonstrating the significance of low HCG levels for predicting preeclampsia, although at a much earlier gestational age than might be practical for spontaneous conceptions [24].

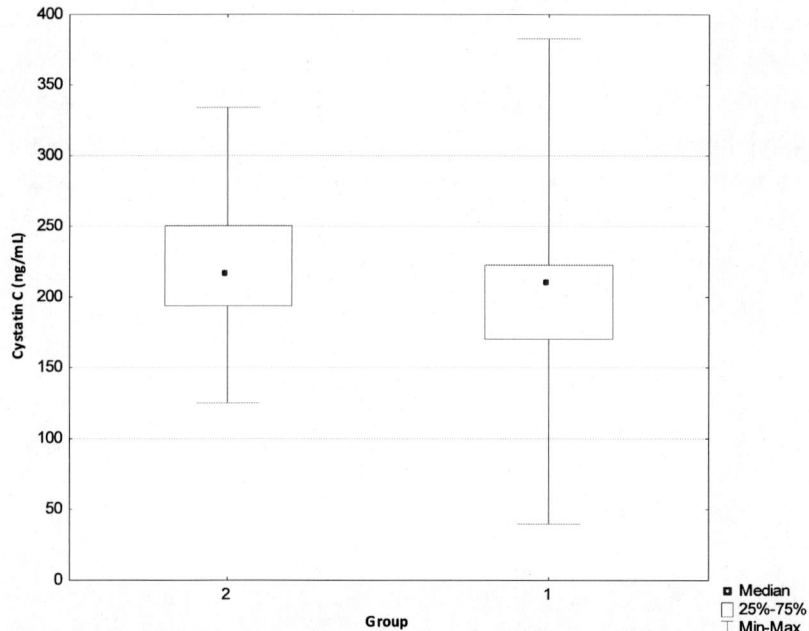

Figure 4. Cystatin C Levels in study groups.

The literature data shows that only combined screening, with the application of maternal factors and serumal ®-HCG, increases the efficiency of identifying severe preeclampsia [25, 26].

According to the design of our study, we made a correlation analysis for each indicator in the group of pregnant women with preeclampsia, the results of which identified statistically meaningful direct correlation of interaction between ADAM12 and RBP4 (p = 0.02), and also between cystatin C and RBP 4 (p = 0.04). For women from the control group we found a meaningful correlation between levels of ADAM12 and RBP4 RBP 4 (p = 0.03). Thus, the received results allowed us to suppose that biomarkers ADAM12 and RBP4 are diagnostically important for early predictors of late-onset preeclampsia of medium severity.

In order to identify the most precise and specific indicators we used the "Decisions trees" method (with the division of drawing into educational and verifying) with the "exhaustive CHAID" construction method, which lead to identifying a meaningful correlation between the group of indicators (RBP4, ADAM12) on the one hand, and the subgroups with preeclampsia and the nominally healthy on the other. Thus, in a case of concentration of RBP4 > 87.90ug/mL, pregnant women should be referred to the "high risk of preeclampsia" group. Additionally, if RBP4 <= 87.90 ug/ml and simultaneously ADAM12 > 2.33ng/ml, pregnant women should also be referred to the "high risk of preeclampsia" group. The forecast of preeclampsia within the framework of this method is done with a sensitivity of 87.5%, and specificity of 85%, with the odds ratio = 39.667 [3.498; 49.83].

CONCLUSION

Preeclampsia, being a threatening pregnancy complication, can be observed in 3% of all pregnant women, and according to the modern national classification, can be divided into early and late forms. The search for parameters, indicating at early stages of gestation the development of late preeclampsia and its morbidity, remains a promising direction for scientific studies. Analysis of the literature data demonstrated that the best predictive meaningfulness belongs to the combination of clinical data and biochemical characteristics. Today the efforts of scientists are being channeled to the development and improvement of multi-factor models of preeclampsia forecasting.

Our study offers the possibility of early predicting for late-onset preeclampsia with medium severity based on a combination of maternal factors only (BMI and MAP). However, a more precise prediction may be made by estimation of biochemical markers RBP4 and ADAM12 levels. The rise of these markers' levels in the case of an increase of BMI and MAP at 11 - 13 weeks screening may points to a high level of possibility of late-onset preeclampsia development (sensitivity rate 87.5% and specificity 85%).

Based on received results we propose the following quantitative criteria and practical recommendations. In the case of MAP > 98 mm HG and BMI > 30.5kg/m2 founded at 11 - 13 weeks of pregnancy, and preeclampsia history in previous pregnancies or chronic arterial hypertension, and chronic pyelonephritis, such pregnant women should be referred to the "high-risk late-onset preeclampsia development" group. If the identified levels of RBP4 is higher than 87.90mkg/ml and ADAM12 is higher than 2.33ng/ml it is advisable to appoint in advance the optimal date of delivery (not later than 34 weeks).

REFERENCES

[1] Duhig, Kate E. and Shennan, Andrew H. 2015. Recent advances in the diagnosis and management of pre-eclampsia. *F1000 Prime Reports*, 7:24. (Duhig 2015, 1) (doi: 10.12703/P7-24).

[2] Gallo, Dahiana, Poon, Leona C., Fernandez, Mariana, Wright, David, Nicolaides, Kypros H. 2014. Prediction of preeclampsia by mean arterial pressure at 11-13 and 20-24 weeks' gestation. *Fetal Diagn. Ther.*, 36(1):28 - 37. (Gallo 2014, 28) (doi: 10.1159/000360287).

[3] Zenclussen, Anna C. 2013. Adaptive immune responses during pregnancy. *Am. J. Reprod. Immunol.*, 69(4):291 - 303. (Zenclussen 2013, 297) (DOI:10,1111/aji.12097).

[4] Park, Hee J., Sung Shin S. and Dong Hyun C. 2015. Combined Screening for Early Detection of Pre-Eclampsia. *Int. J. Mol. Sci.*, 16:17952 - 17974. (Hee 2015, 17953). (doi:10.3390/ijms160817952).

[5] Bateman, Brian T., Bansil, Pooja, Hernandez-Diaz, Sonia, Mhyre, Jill M., Callaghan, William M., Kuklina, Elena V. 2012. Prevalence, trends, and outcomes of chronic hypertension: a nationwide sample of delivery admissions. *Am. J. Obstet. Gynecol.*, 206(2):134 - 8. (Bateman 2012, 135) (doi:10.1016/j.ajog.2011.10.878).

[6] Bakker, Rachel, Steegers, Eric A., Hofman, Albert and Jaddoe, Vincent. 2011. Blood pressure in different gestational trimesters, fetal growth, and the risk of adverse birth outcomes: the generation R study. *Am. J. Epidemiol.*, 174(7):797 - 806. (Bakker 2011, 805) (doi: 10.1093/aje/kwr151).

[7] Baschat, Ahmet A., Magder, Laurence S., Doyle, Lauren E., Atlas, Robert O., Jenkins, Chuka B., Bilizer, Miriam G. 2014. Prediction of preeclampsia utilizing the first trimester screening examination. *Am. J. Obstet. Gynecol.*, 211(5):514. e1-7. (Baschat 2014) (doi: https://doi.org/10.1016/j.ajog.2014.04.018).

[8] Sung, Kyung Uk, Roh Jeong A, Eoh Kyung J., Kim Eui H. 2017. Maternal serum placental growth factor and pregnancy-associated plasma protein A measured in the first trimester as parameters of subsequent preeclampsia and small-for-gestational-age infants: A prospective observational study. *Obstet. Gynecol. Sci.*, 60(2):154 - 62. (Sung 2017, 155) (doi: 10.5468/ogs.2017.60.2.154).

[9] Giguere, Yves, Masse´, Jacques, Theriault, Sebastien, Bujold, Emmanuel, Laford, Julie, Rosseau, Francois and Forest, Jean C. 2015. Screening for preeclampsia early in pregnancy: performance of a multivariable model combining clinical characteristics and biochemical markers. *BJOG*, 122(3): 402 - 10. (Giguere 2015, 402, 406). (doi: 10.1111/1471-0528.13050).

[10] Myatt, Leslie, Clifton, Rebecca G., Roberts, James M., Spong, Catherine Y., Hauth, John C., Varner, Michael W. et al. 2012. Eunice Kennedy Shriver National Institute of Child Health and Human Development [NICHD] Maternal-Fetal Medicine Units [MFMU] Network. First-trimester prediction of preeclampsia in nulliparous women at low risk. *Obstet. Gynecol.*, 119(6): 1234 - 42. (Myatt 2012, 1235). (doi:10.1097/AOG.0b013e3182571669).

[11] Matwejew, Cowans, Nicholas J., Stamatopoulou, Anastasia, Spencer, Kevin, von Kaisenberg, Constantine S. 2010. Maternal serum ADAM-12 as a potential marker for different adverse pregnancy outcomes. *Fetal Diagn. Ther.*, 27(1): 32 - 9. (Matwejew 2010, 32). (doi: 10.1159/000275669).

[12] Wright, David, Syngelaki, Argyro, Akolekar, Ranjit, Poon, Leona C., Nicolaides, Kypros H. 2015. Competing risks model in screening for preeclampsia by maternal characteristics and medical history. *Am. J. Obstet. Gynecol.*, 213(1): 1 - 10. (Wright 2015, 1 - 2). (doi.org/ 10.1016/j.ajog.2015.02.018).

[13] Zhang, Zhenyu, He Jin. 2015. Risk factors of recurrent preeclampsia and its relation to maternal and offspring outcome. *Zhejiang Da Xue Xue Bao Yi Xue Ban,* 2015; 44(3):258 - 63. (Zhang 2015, 258).

[14] Itoh, Hiroaki, Kanayama, Naohiro. 2014. Obesity and risk of preeclampsia. *Med. J. Obstet. Gynecol.*, 2(2): 1024. (Iton 2014, 1 - 5).

[15] Baeten, Jared M., Bukusi, Elizabeth A., Lambe, Mats. 2001. Pregnancy complications and outcomes among overweight and obese nulliparous women. *Am. J. Public Health*, 91:436 - 440. (Baeten 2001, 437). (doi:10.2105/ajph.91.3.436).

[16] Iacobelli, Silvia, Bonsante, Francesco, Robillard, Pierre-Yves. 2017. Comparison of risk factors and perinatal outcomes in early onset and late onset preeclampsia: A cohort-based study in Reunion Island. *J. Reprod. Immunol.*, 123: 12 - 16. (Iacobelli 2017, 12) (doi.org/ 10.1016/j.jri.2017.08.005).

[17] Vodneva, Dariya N., Shmakov, Roman G., Shchegolev, Aleksandr I. 2013 Role of markers for trophoblast invasion in the development of

preeclampsia and tumor progression. *Akusherstvo i Ginekologiya/ Obstetrics and Gynecology*, 11: 9 - 12. (in Russian).

[18] Mendola, Pauline, Ghassabian, Akhgar, Mills, James L., Zhang, Cuilin, Tsai, Michael Y., Liu Aiyi, Yeung, Edwina H. 2017. Retinol-binding protein 4 and lipids prospectively measured during early to mid-pregnancy in relation to preeclampsia and preterm birth risk. *Am. J. Hypertens.*, 30(6): 569 - 76. (Mendola 2017, 573). (doi: 10.1093/ajh/hpx020).

[19] Al-Kholy, Adel, Abadier, Mamdouh Z., Rageh, Ebrahem M., El-Kallaf, Hany. 2010. Serum levels of placental growth factor and retinol-binding protein-4 in pregnancy-induced hypertensive women. *J. Am. Sci.*, 6(12):448 - 55. (Al-Kholy 2010, 448).

[20] Stepan, Holger, Ebert, Thomas, Schrey, Susanne, Reisenbüchler, Constanze, Blüher, Matthias, Stumvoll, Michael, Kratzsch, Jürgen, Tönnessen, Patricia, Faber, Renaldo, Fasshauer, Mathias. 2009. Preliminary report: Serum levels of RBP-4 in preeclampsia. *Metabolism*, 58:275 - 277. (Stepan 2009, 277). (doi.org/10.1016/j.metabol.2008.10.001).

[21] Kristensen, Karl, Larsson, Irene, Hansson, Stefan. 2007. Increased cystatin C expression in the preeclamptic placenta. *Mol. Hum. Reprod.*, 13:189 - 195. (Kristensen 2007, 192 - 194). (doi:10.1093/molehr/gal111).

[22] Thilaganathan, Basky, Ralph, Elizabeth, Papageorghiou, Aris T., Melchiorre, Karen, Sheldon, Joanna. 2009. Raised maternal serum cystatin C: an early pregnancy marker for preeclampsia. *Reprod. Sci.*, 16: 788 - 793. (Thilaganathan 2009, 788). (doi.org/10.1177/1933719109336618).

[23] Asvold, Bjørn O., Vatten, Lars J., Tanbo, Tom G., Eskild, Anne. 2014. Concentrations of human chorionic gonadotrophin in very early pregnancy and subsequent preeclampsia: a cohort study. *Hum. Reprod.*, 29(6):1153 - 1160. (Asvold 2014, 1153). (doi.org/10.1093/humrep/deu068).

[24] Rabie, Nader Z., Magann, Everett F. 2014. Human chronic gonadotropin concentrations in very early pregnancy and subsequent

preeclampsia. *Women's Health,* (Lond Engl). 10(5):483 - 485. (Rabie 2014, 485).

[25] Keikkala, Elina, Vuorela, Piia, Laivuori, Hannele M., Romppanen, Jarkko, Heinonen, Seppo T., Stenman, Ulf Håkan E. 2013. First trimester hyperglycosylated human chorionic gonadotrophin in serum–a marker of early-onset preeclampsia. *Placenta,* 34(11):1059 - 1065. (Keikkala 2013б 1059). (doi.org/10.1016/ j.placenta.2013. 08.006).

[26] Androutsopoulos, Georgios, Gkogkos, Panagiotis, Decavalas, Georgios. 2013. Mid-trimester maternal serum HCG and alpha fetal protein levels: clinical significance and prediction of adverse pregnancy outcome//*Int. J. Endocrinol. Metab.,* 11(2):102 - 106. (Androutsopoulos 2013, 102). (doi: 10.5812/ijem. 5014).

Reviewed by: Professor Vitaly Bezhenar
Head of the Department of Obstetrics, Gynecology and Neonatology
Head of the Department of Obstetrics, Gynecology and Reproductology
Head of Obstetrics and Gynecology Hospital Scientific Secretary of the Scientific Council of the Pavlov State Medical University Ministry of Health of Russia
Chief Obstetrician-Gynecologist of the Ministry of Health of Russia in North-Western Federal Region
197022 • 6-8 Lev Tolstoy str. • Saint Petersburg • Russia. Tel/Fax: +7 812 3290333. Mob. +79219351173, +79315391966. Phone: +7812338-67-44. e-mail: bez-vitaly@yandex.ru.

BIOGRAPHICAL SKETCH

Svetlana Dubrovina

Affiliation: Obstetrics & Gynecology
Education: Rostov Medical Institute

Business Address:
Mechnikova 43, Rostov-on-Don, Russia
Professional Appointments: the main scientific researcher of Rostov Scientific Research Institute of Obstetrics and Pediatrics of Rostov State University
Honors: PhD of Medicine, Professor
Publications from the Last 3 Years:
CV & list of last publications are available upon request

In: Preeclampsia
Editor: Torsten Nacht

ISBN: 978-1-53617-116-7
© 2020 Nova Science Publishers, Inc.

Chapter 2

PREECLAMPSIA PATHOGENESIS

Nese Colcimen[*], MD, PhD
Department of Medicine, Van Yuzuncu Yil University,
Van, Turkey

ABSTRACT

Preeclampsia is usually defined as new-onset hypertension and proteinuria diagnosed at 20th gestational week or after. Preeclampsia is one of the leading causes of maternal and infant mortality worldwide. It is important to clarify its pathogenesis for its treatment and prevention. This chapter summarized some theories suggested to explain the pathogenesis of preeclampsia. The pathogenesis of preeclampsia has not yet been fully clarified and it remains a disease of theories. Furthermore, as it is a human-specific disease, the lack of one-on-one animal modeling and many other factors contribute to poor understanding of the disease pathophysiology. For this reason, continuous efforts have been made and new theories have been put forth to explain the disease pathophysiology. New data have revealed the unknowns and guide our understanding about the mechanism of the multifactorial pathogenesis of the disease. Our hope is that the accumulation of knowledge on the subject will clarify the pathogenesis of the disease and make us reach a definitive conclusion in the treatment and prevention of the disease in the near future.

---

[*] Corresponding Author: colcimennese@hotmail.com.

Keywords: pathogenesis, placenta, preeclampsia

Preeclampsia is one of the leading causes of maternal and infant mortality worldwide. Preeclampsia is a multisystem disorder of pregnancy that is usually defined as new-onset hypertension and proteinuria diagnosed at 20th gestational week or after [1]. Currently, however, preeclampsia is defined as a 2-stage disease where Stage 1 involves reduced placental perfusion and abnormal implantation, and stage 2 defines maternal syndrome [2]. The pathogenesis of preeclampsia has not yet been fully clarified and it remains a disease of theories. Furthermore, as it is a human-specific disease, the lack of one-on-one animal modeling and many other factors contribute to a poor understanding of the disease pathophysiology.

Theories associated with the pathogenesis of preeclampsia are the following:

1-Abnormal Placental Development
2-Immunological Factors
3-Genetic Factors
4-Metabolic and Nutritional Factors
5-Systemic Endothelial Dysfunction
6-Inflammation
7- Oxidative Stress
8-Renin Angiotensin system imbalance

1. Abnormal Placental Development

The placenta plays an important role in the development and remission of preeclampsia. The fact that the disease is treated with separation of the placenta and that the disease is more severe in women with hydatid mole containing no fetus both prove this hypothesis [3].

1.1. Abnormal Structure of Spiral Arteries

The transformation of the spiral arteries into the uteroplacental arteries is probably a physiological change that begins at the end of the first trimester and is completed at 18-20 weeks of gestation [4]. This change takes place in two stages. The first stage involves trophoblastic wave invasion. In the first trimester, the decidual segments of the spiral arteries and the second trophoblastic wave invasion change the myometrial (myometrium 1/3 inner layer) segments of the spiral arteries in the 2nd trimester. As a result of these changes, the spiral arteries are transformed from small muscular arteries of 15-20 micron in diameter into low-capacity high-capacity vessels with a diameter of 300-500 micron. Thus, this region of the uterus reduces resistance to current in the intervillous distance, becomes high-current, augmenting the feto-maternal cell traffic. These events are usually completed by 20th week, resulting in loss of mucoblastic properties of the radial arteries and insensitivity to vasoactive (vasopressor) agents. In preeclampsia, however, the response to vasopressors increases due to an impairment of this change. Previous studies using placental bed biopsies have shown that in normal pregnancies cytotrophoblastic cells invade spiral arteries whose muscular tissue has been shown disappear completely and lumen dilated. Additionally, it has been reported that there is no mural thrombus and fibrinoid storage in the endothelial layer. In preeclampsia, these physiological events occur only in the periphery and the decidual part of the spiral arteries. The veins do not enter the section within the myometrium; incomplete remodeling occurs; smooth muscle and elastic layers of the spiral arteries remain; so, the invasion and dilatation of the vessel does not occur [5]. As a result, in preeclamptic pregnancies fetoplacental blood flow does not increase progressively with pregnancy and fetal growth retardation occurs [6, 7]. It is not known exactly why there is no proper placental structure in some pregnant women, but some vascular, environmental, immunological, and genetic factors are thought to play a role [8].

1.2. Defective Trophoblastic Differentiation

Defective differentiation of trophoblasts is one of the events that cause problematic invasion of spiral arteries [9]. The endothelial invasion process involves changes in the expression of molecules from different classes such as trophoblast differentiation, cytokines, metalloproteinases, extracellular matrix molecules, adhesion molecules and Ib class Human Leukocyte Antigen-G (HLA-G) [10]. As a result of the problems in differentiation during endothelial invasion, adhesion and extracellular matrix molecules containing cytokines cause problems in metalloproteinases and Ib class HLA-G levels [11]. Thus, intercellular communication is impaired. In this process, some basic morphological changes occur in trophoblasts. The trophoblast invasion during normal differentiation alter adhesion molecule expression to the endothelial cell shape (integrin, alpha1 / beta1, alfav / beta3, and VE-cadherin) from the epithelial cell-specific (integrin alpha 6 / beta 1, alfav / beta5 and E-cadherin), a process which is called pseudo-vasculogenesis [10]. The trophoblasts obtained from preeclamptic women do not show adhesion molecule expression or pseudo-vasculogenesis [4], which suggests that impaired placentation and accompanying ischemia are primary events leading to the placental release of soluble substances, which cause systemic endothelial dysfunction resulting in preeclampsia.

1.3. Hypoperfusion, Hypoxia and Ischemia

Hypoperfusion in preeclampsia is the result and cause of abnormal placental development. In animal samples where preeclampsia is partly modeled, decreased uteroplacental blood flow, vascular failure related medical conditions (hypertension, diabetes mellitus, systemic lupus erythematosus, kidney harvests, acquired and hereditary thrombophilia) increase the risk of abnormal placentation and preeclampsia. The increased risk of preeclampsia in women surviving high altitude and cases with increased placental mass but unchanged placental flow resulting in relative ischemia (hydatid mole, hydrops fetalis, diabetes mellitus, twin pregnancy) support this theory. Hypo-perfused, ischemic placenta leads to the release of various factors that disrupt maternal endothelial cell function to systemic circulation, leading to the emergence of characteristic signs of preeclampsia [10]. Hypoperfusion and hypoperfusion-reperfusion injury is a powerful stimulant for endoplasmic reticulum (ER). When ER stress response cannot protect cellular hemostasis and prevent oxidative and inflammatory stress, apoptosis/necrosis of the syncitio-trophoblastic layer occurs [12].

Late placental changes consistent with ischemia include atherosis, thrombosis, sclerotic stenosis of arterioles, fibrinoid necrosis, and placental infarction. While these lesions are not identical in all pregnant women, there are related to preeclampsia severity [13].

2. IMMUNOLOGICAL FACTORS

The hypothesis that immunological factors may contribute to abnormal placental development is based on the observation that pre-exposure to paternal/fetal antigens is protective against preeclampsia. This theory supports the observations that preeclampsia prevalence is increased in nullipara women, frequency of partner changes is reduced, the frequency barrier method as a contraceptive method is increased, and pregnancy formed of assisted reproductive techniques [10].

Chemotaxis and adhesion functions of polymorphonuclear leukocytes gradually decrease starting from the second trimester in normal pregnancy. This immunological suppression in pregnant women partially explains the improvement occurring in autoimmune diseases and an easier to catch of infections. In preeclampsia, blocking antibodies are decreased, and cytokines and neutrophils are activated [13].

The trophoblast cells must establish close tissue contact with allogenic cells for the invasion of the decidua with intensive leukocyte infiltration and subsequent arterial change. They do not produce classical HLA mRNA or HLA protein in extra-villous trophoblasts (EVT) membranes and thus do not show immunological rejection reaction. Although the classical class I HLA antigens are absent, cytotrophoblasts express non-classical HLA G, HLA-C, and HLA-E antigens [4]. Non-polymorphic HLA-G plays an important role in the protection of trophoblasts from cytotoxic effects induced by natural killer (NK) cells. Besides, NK cells activated by HLA-G are very effective in important vascular changes [14, 15].

NK cells are the major immune cell type in decidua in early pregnancy and mid-secretory phase of menstruation. (%70-75). As the pregnancy progresses, the NK cell number gradually increases. Decidual NK cells accumulate around the extra-villous cytotrophoblasts and near the uterine spiral arteries, indicating that they play an important role in the modulation of vascular remodeling and trophoblast invasion [16]. Based on this, one of the most important products of NK cells, Interferon-gamma (IFN-gamma), was investigated. In the experiments, IFN-gamma derived from uterine NK cells has also been shown to be necessary in the pregnancy-induced spiral artery modification. IFN-gamma release stimulates genes that stimulate alpha2-macroglobulin release. Alfa2-macroglobulin also regulates proteases, cytokines, and other mediators that are effective in vascular dilation [14]. The most effective cells in adaptation to immune response are T cells, with significant absence of T-cell interaction in preeclampsia, leading to immune maladaptation [15]. The balance between the Th1 / Th2 immune response is mandatory for the continuation of normal pregnancy. In normal pregnancies, the lymphocyte balance is in favor of Th2 / suppressor T-helper. This balance suppresses the negative effects of cytotoxic Th1 / pro-inflammatory-T-helper, allowing for maternal immune tolerance to the fetal allograft. In preeclampsia, the activation of Th1 cells is greater than Th2 cells and preeclamptic patients have higher levels of cytokine secretion than Th1 lymphocytes. These cytokines cause placental formation and endothelial dysfunction leading to preeclampsia [17, 18].

An important development in immunoassay theory in preeclampsia is the detection of increased antibodies to angiotensin AT-1 receptors. These antibodies release intracellular calcium and thereby increase the production of plasminogen activator 1 and reduce trophoblast invasion in preeclampsia. However, more studies are needed on this antibody [4].

3. GENETIC FACTORS

Genetic predisposition has an important role in the pathogenesis of preeclampsia, but the genetic transition pattern has not been fully demonstrated. The risk of preeclampsia in the presence of preeclampsia in the mother and sister increases by 2-5-fold [9].

fms-like tyrosine kinase (Flt-1, also known as vascular endothelial growth factor receptor 1 (VEGFR-1)) and Soluble Flt-1 (sFlt-1) genes are transported on chromosome 13. Fetuses carrying one more copy of this chromosome (such as trisomy 13) produce more of the products of this gene than normal. The risk of preeclampsia in mothers with trisomy 13 fetuses is increased with respect to all trisomies and control group pregnancies. In addition, the rate of circulating sFlt-1 / Placental growth factor (PlGF) was significantly increased in these pregnant subjects, contributing to an increased risk of preeclampsia [10].

Multifactorial inheritance has also been shown to be involved in studies [20]. It has also been found that the genes related to obesity constitute more preeclampsia risk than other factors [21].

Four gene loci responsible for preeclampsia were detected in genome studies. These are 2p12, 2p25, 10q22, and 9p13 [22].

No single genetic mechanism specific for preeclampsia has been demonstrated.

4. METABOLIC AND NUTRITIONAL FACTORS

Salt and protein restriction, zinc, magnesium, fish oil administration, diuretic and other antihypertensive drugs, aspirin and heparin use were evaluated in studies. However, the treatments were minimally effective or ineffective due to a limited number of cases [23, 24].

There are many studies investigating the relationship between calcium intake and hypertension in the diet. Calcium decreases blood pressure by decreasing vascular sensitivity against angiotensin during pregnancy [13]. However, different results were obtained in different studies.

Vitamin C and vitamin E levels decrease significantly in preeclampsia. Decrease of these vitamins causes oxidative stress. Vitamin E breaks the lipid peroxidation chain by inhibiting NAD (P) H Oxidase in placental tissue. Vitamin C also helps convert Vitamin E into a biologically used form. It has been shown in studies that the combined use of vitamin C and E has beneficial effects [25]. Due to its antioxidant effects, beta-carotene studies are available.

High body mass index increases the risk of preeclampsia. Obesity probably leads to susceptibility to preeclampsia by inducing chronic inflammation and endothelial dysfunction [4].

5. SYSTEMIC ENDOTHELIAL DYSFUNCTION

Vascular endothelial damage and vasospasm play an important role in the pathogenesis of preeclampsia. The venous endothelial layer acts as a mechanical and metabolic barrier, regulates capillary transport, directs the activity of smooth muscles around the vein, and functions in hemostasis [26]. Healthy vascular endothelium secretes some mediators such as nitric oxide, adenosine, which inhibit platelet activation and therefore adhesion to the endothelium [27].

Maternal endothelial dysfunction is common in preeclampsia and explains all clinical signs of the disease [28]. Increased pressor response, nitrite oxide, endothelin, prostaglandins, vascular growth factor, genetic predisposition, inflammatory and immunological factors are responsible for the development of vascular endothelial damage and vasospasm and showed a close relationship with endothelial cell activation. Inadequate placental blood flow induces the release of hormones and chemical agents, especially those that damage the endothelium. These include Von Willebrand antigen, cellular fibronectin, soluble tissue factor, soluble E-selectin, platelet derived growth factor, and endothelin [3].

Nitric oxide (NO) is a vasodilating agent that is synthesized by NO synthase from L-arginine in endothelial cells. The absence or decreased concentration of NO in pregnancy-induced hypertensive diseases is thought to play a role [26]. Endothelium-induced vasodilator effective prostacyclin production also decreases in preeclampsia [4].

Endothelin is a potent vasoconstrictor that is secreted from the vascular endothelium [29]. In preeclampsia, the production of vasoconstrictors such as endothelin and thromboxane is increased [4].

Increased vascular reactivity to angiotensin 2 occurs [10].

In placentation, angiogenesis is necessary to establish a suitable vascular network to provide the fetus with oxygen and nutrition. For a normal placental development, there should be a balance between proangiogenic (VEGF, PIGF) and antiangiogenic (sFlt-1) factors. Systemic endothelial dysfunction occurs if the production of antiangiogenic factors increases and that balance is disrupted [4].

Vascular endothelial growth factor (VEGF) is a glycoprotein found in the human placenta. It is important in vasculo-genesis and vascular permeability control. It is necessary for endothelial stability and plays an important role in the pathogenesis of preeclampsia. The level of VEGF in preeclampsia was found to be high and a relationship between VEGF and uteroplacental vessel resistance has been shown [30].

The placental growth factor (PIGF) is another member of the VEGF family and is predominantly synthesized from the placenta. It also binds to the VEGFR-1 receptor [4].

sFlt1 binds to VEGF and PIGF in circulation and inhibits their reaction with endogenous receptors and antagonizes them. In preeclampsia, the level of sFlt1 increases in maternal circulation [3].

The presence of transforming growth factor beta (TGF-β) such as sFlt1 negatively affects trophoblast invasion. TGF-β decreases at 9 weeks in normal pregnancy, which initiates cytotrophoblast invasion. TGF-β increases in preeclamptic placentas [3].

Tumor necrosis factor alpha (TNF-α) levels are high in patients with preeclampsia. The main place of production is the placenta. The reason for high levels of TNF-α expression of the placenta is hypoxia or hypoxia-reoxygenation. TNF-α in the blood is in direct contact with maternal endothelial cells in in vivo medium and causes damage to them [31].

6. INFLAMMATION

Preeclampsia is a systemic inflammatory disease that causes damage to maternal organs (liver, kidney, lung, and central nervous system). It has been hypothesized that circulating cytotrophoblast debris contributes to maternal inflammation and some signs of the syndrome. Trophoblastic debris and microparticles in normal pregnancies are proinflammatory, and this process has been found to be augmented in preeclampsia [10]. In preeclampsia, hypoxia, inflammation or oxidative stress in the placenta leads to necrosis or aponeurosis instead of apoptosis in trophoblasts. Necrotic trophoblasts released into the maternal circulation are phagocytosed by dendritic cells, which secrete cytokines such as TNF- α, IL-12, and IFN-c [32]. In addition, the microparticles carry antiangiogenic proteins such as soluble fms-like tyrosine kinase (sFlt-1) and soluble endoglin (sEng) [10]. sFlt-1 binds to VEGF and PlGF which play a role in maintaining the integrity of vascular endothelin and neutralizing their angiogenic effect. sEng is anti-angiogenic agent, whose angiogenic effects are antagonized by TGF-β binding. sFlt-1 and sEng have synergistic effects when co-administered. In preeclampsia, sFlt-1 and sEng levels are increased whereas VEGF and PlGF levels are decreased. These alterations are correlated with the severity of the disease [33].

Endothelial cell dysfunction occurring in preeclampsia is explained by the hypothesis of "generalized irregularity status of normal, generalized maternal intravascular maladaptation of pregnancy." In this hypothesis, preeclampsia is considered as a disease caused by overexcitation of active leukocytes in the maternal circulation. There are plenty of cells in deciduas that can secrete harmful substances when activated. Aberrant infiltration of antigen presenting cells (APC), macrophages, and dendritic cells have been shown in preeclamptic decidua. During pregnancy, a number of cytokines have been shown to be expressed in addition to immune cells from both decidual cells and extra-villous cytotrophoblast cells [16].

Cytokines are regulatory molecules that have effects on cell functions. Balanced and properly structured cytokine expression in the cells located in the Materno-fetal junction is necessary for normal formation and development of the placenta. Cytokines also regulate endothelial function. The two most important factors involved in the pathogenesis of preeclampsia are placenta formation and widespread endothelial damage. For this reason, there may be a significant link between cytokine release, occurrence of disorders and imbalances, and the emergence of preeclampsia [34].

Damage-associated molecular patterns (DAMPs) are pro-inflammatory intracellular molecules released upon cell stress or injury. They include High-mobility Group Box Protein 1(HMGB1), Heat Shock Protein 70 (HSP70), S100B, Advanced Glycation End Products (AGEs), Cell Free ATP, Actin, Haemoglobin, and Fetal DNA. They activate maternal immune cells through receptors such as toll-like (TRLs) and receptor for advanced glycation end products (RAGE), resulting in potent systemic inflammation and endothelial dysfunction [35].

7. OXIDATIVE STRESS

Pregnancy is an oxidative stress condition. With the explosion of oxidative stress in the first trimester, blood flow to the intervillous area is provided. An insufficient antioxidant defense system was observed in preeclampsia during later stages of pregnancy, which is thought to cause changes in trophoblast apoptosis and placental vascular reactivity [36].

The reason for the increase of placenta-induced oxidative stress is hypoxia and ischemia-reperfusion type damage caused by the problems in spiral artery structure. Free radicals resulting from oxidative stress lead to lipid peroxidation, protein and DNA damage. Free radicals increase the apoptosis of trophoblasts, and this finding has been found in placenta examination of preeclamptic pregnancies. In addition, free radicals entering systemic circulation cause lipid peroxidation and extensive oxidative damage in the vascular endothelium throughout the body [37]. This reduces NO's endothelial production and disrupts prostaglandin balance, which we have mentioned above as a result of endothelial dysfunction.

Other results of oxidative stress include activation of microvascular coagulation (thrombocytopenia); production of lipid-loaded macrophages (foam cells) which are characteristic of atherosclerosis; and increase in capillary permeability (edema, proteinuria) [30, 38]. Oxidative stress modifies proteins and lipids. Maternal LDL is converted to oxidized LDL. Oxidized LDL binds to Lectin-like oxidized LDL receptor-1 (LOX-1). Placenta and systemic LOX-1 expression are increased in preeclampsia, which leads to endothelial dysfunction and increased oxidative stress [39].

8. RENIN ANGIOTENSIN SYSTEM IMBALANCE

The renin-angiotensin-aldosterone axis is suppressed in preeclampsia. Angiotensin and aldosterone are increased in normal pregnancy. In preeclampsia, vascular sensitivity increases to other vasoconstrictive agents and angiotensin II. Plasma renin / aldosterone is relatively suppressed in preeclampsia compared with normal pregnancies [3]. It has been found that angiotensin levels, renin levels and angiotensin converting enzyme mRNA expression are higher in preeclamptic pregnancies compared to normal pregnancies [40]. In preeclamptic women, thromboxane is elevated while prostacyclin and prostaglandin E2 decrease. As a result, vasoconstriction and susceptibility to infused angiotensin II ensues. While normal pregnant women are not easily affected by the infusion of vasopressors, preeclamptic pregnant women show increased vascular sensitivity to the vasopressors, especially angiotensin [30]. Such angiotensin II hypersensitivity in preeclampsia is thought to be secondary to active and bonded angiotensin receptor autoantibodies. Angiotensin II receptor autoantibodies may contribute to inadequate placental invasion of syncytio-trophoblasts by causing endothelial damage and the production of antiangiogenic factors [3]. The exact mechanism by which prostaglandin and similar substances regulate vascular reactivity during pregnancy is unknown. Compared with normal pregnancies, preeclampsia is characterized by significantly reduced prostacyclin levels, significantly increased thromboxane A2, and vasoconstriction [26].

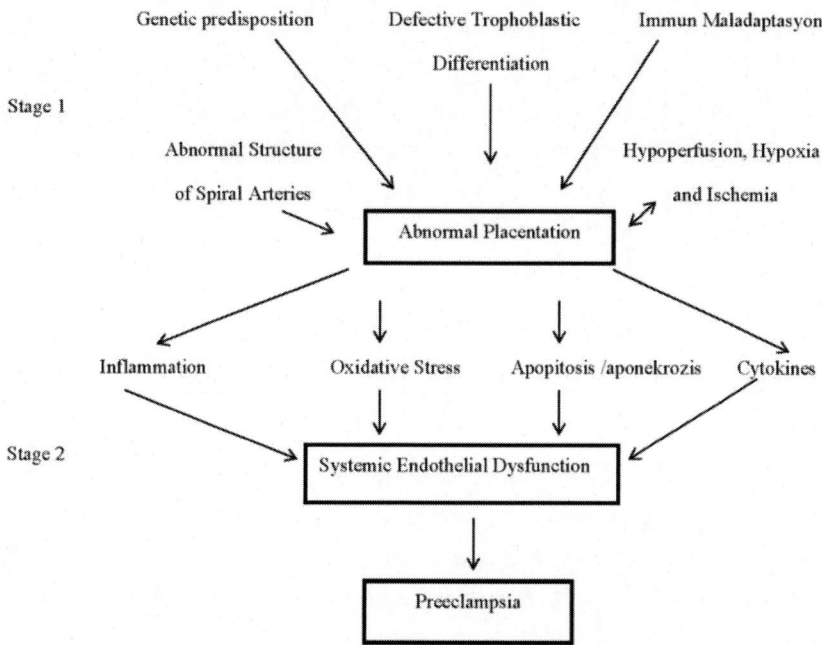

Figure 1. Summary of the pathogenesis of preeclampsia.

REFERENCES

[1] Atallah, A., Lecarpentier, E., Goffinet, F., Doret-Dion, M., Gaucherand, P., Tsatsaris, V. (2017). Aspirin for Prevention of Preeclampsia. *Drugs,* 77 (XVII): 1819-1831.
[2] Roberts, J. M., Hubel, C. A. (2009). The two stage model of preeclampsia: variations on the theme. *Placenta,* 30: 32-37.
[3] Young, B. C., Levine, R. J., Karumanchi, S. A. (2010). Pathogenesis of preeclampsia. *Annu. Rev. Pathol.* 5: 173-192.

[4] Karumanchi, S. A., Lim, K. H., August, P. (opened. Jun 06, 2018). *Preeclampsia: Pathogenesis.* Section Editor: Vincenzo Berghella, www.uptodate.com ©2019 UpToDate. Date

[5] Staff, A. C., Benton, S .J., von Dadelszen, P., Roberts, J. M., Taylor, R. N., Powers, R. W., Charnock-Jones, D. S., Redman, C.W. (2013). Redefining preeclampsia using placenta-derived biomarkers. *Hypertension*, 61 (V): 932-942.

[6] Kaufmann, P., Black, S., Huppertz, B. (2003). Endovascular trophoblast invasion: Implications for the pathogenesis of intrauterine growth retardation and preeclampsia. *Biol. Reprod.* 69 (I): 1-7.

[7] Ong, S. S., Baker, P. N., Mayhev, T. M., Dunn, W. R. (2005). Remodeling of myometrial radial arteries in preeclampsia. *Am. J. Obstet. Gynecol.* 192 (II): 572-579.

[8] Ilekis, J. V., Reddy, U. M., Roberts, J. M. (2007). Preeclampsia--a pressing problem: an executive summary of a National Institute of Child Health and Human Development workshop. *Reprod. Sci.* 14 (VI): 508-523.

[9] Huppertz, B. (2008). Placental origins of preeclampsia: challenging the current hypothesis. *Hypertension,* 51 (IV): 970-975.

[10] Sevinc, A. (2016). *Histopathological examination of placenta in pregnancies associated with placentation disorder.* Published Ph.D. Thesis, Osmangazi University, Eskisehir.

[11] Lim, K. H., Zhou, Y., Janatpour, M., McMaster, M., Bass, K., Chun, S. H., Fisher, S. J. (1997). Human cytotrophoblast differentiation/invasion is abnormal in pre-eclampsia. *Am. J. Pathol.* 151 (VI): 1809-1818.

[12] Burton, G. J., Yung, H. W., Cindrova-Davies, T., Charnock-Jones, D. S. (2009). Placental endoplasmic reticulum stress and oxidative stress in the pathophysiology of unexplained intrauterine growth restriction and early onset preeclampsia. *Placenta*, 30: 43-48.

[13] Goktepe, H. (2011). *Investigation of fetal umbilical artery, ductus venosus, middle cerebral artery doppler findings in preeclamptic patients.* Published Ph.D. Thesis, Selcuk University, Konya.

[14] Croy, B. A., He, H., Esadeg, S., Wei, Q., McCartney, D., Zhang, J., Borzychowski, A., Ashkar, A. A., Black, G. P., Evans, S. S., Chantakru, S., Van den Heuvel, M., Paffaro, V. A. Jr., Yamada, A. T. (2003). Uterine natural killer cells; insight into their cellular and molecular biology from mouse modelling. *Reproduction*, 126 (II): 149-160.
[15] Van der Meer, A., Lukassen, H. G., Van Lierop, M. J., Wijnands, F., Mosselman, S., Braat, D. D., Joosten, I. (2004). Membrane-bound HLA-G activates proliferation and interferon-gamma production by uterine natural killer cells. *Mol. Hum. Reprod.* 10 (III): 189-195.
[16] Yeh, C. C., Chao, K. C., Huang, S. J. (2013). Innate immunity, decidual cells, and preeclampsia. *Reprod. Sci.* 20 (IV): 339-353.
[17] Gezginc, K., Yazici, F. (2013). Hypertensive diseases of pregnancy. Review. *Medical Research Journal*, 11: 1-9.
[18] Cudihy, D., Lee, R. V. (2009). The pathophysiology of preeclampsia: current clinical concepts. *J. Obstet. Gynaecol.* 29 (VII): 576-582.
[19] Cnattingius, S., Reilly, M., Pawitan, Y., Lichtenstein, P. (2004). Maternal and fetal genetic factors account for most of familial aggregation of preeclampsia: a population-based Swedish cohort study. *Am. J. Med. Genet.* A, 130: 365-371.
[20] Kilpatrick, D. C., Liston, W. A., Gibson, F., Livingstone, J. (1989). Association between susceptibility to pre-eclampsia within families and HLA DR4. *Lancet,* 2: 1063-1065.
[21] Reimer, T., Koczan, D., Gerber, B., Richter, D., Thiesen, H. J., Friese, K. (2002). Microarray analysis of differentially expressed genes in placental tissue of pre-eclampsia: up-regulation of obesityrelatedgenes. *Mol. Hum. Reprod.* 8 (VII): 674-680.
[22] Laivuori, H., Lahermo, P., Ollikainen, V., Widen, E., Häivä-Mällinen, L., Sundström, H., Laitinen, T., Kaaja, R., Ylikorkala, O., Kere, J. (2003). Susceptibility loci for preeclampsia on chromosomes 2p25 and 9p13 in finnish families. *Am. J. Hum. Genet.* 72 (I): 168-177.

[23] Magee, L. A., Duley, L. (2003). Oral beta-blockers for mild to moderate hypertension during pregnancy. *Cochrane Database Syst. Rev.* 3: CD002863.
[24] Holmes, V. A., McCance, D. R. (2005). Could antioxidant supplementation prevent pre-eclampsia? *Proc. Nutr. Soc.* 64 (IV): 491-501.
[25] Gupta, S., Agarwal, A., Sharma, R. K. (2005). The role of placental oxidative stress and lipid peroxidation in preeclampsia. *Obstet. Gynecol. Surv.* 60 (XII): 807-816.
[26] D'Anna, R., Baviera, G., Corrado, F., Crisafulli, A., Ientile, R., Buemi, M., Squadrito, F. (2004). Neurokinin B and nitric oxide plasma levels in pre-eclampsia and isolated intrauterine growth restriction. *BJOG*, 111: 1046-1050.
[27] Sahin, S., Ozakpinar, O. B., Eroglu, M., Tetik, S. (2014). Platelet in preeclampsia: function and role in the inflammation. *Journal of Marmara Univesity Institute of Health Sciences*, 4: 111-116.
[28] Siddiqui, I. A., Jaleel, A., Tamimi, W., Al Kadri, H. M. F. (2010). Role of oxidative stress in the pathogenesis of preeclampsia. *Arch. Gynecol. Obstet.* 282 (V): 469-474.
[29] Aydin, S., Benian, A., Madazli, R., Uludag, S., Uzun, H., Kaya, S. (2004). Plasma malondialdehyde, superoxide dismutase, sE-selectin, fibronectin, endothelin-1 and nitric oxide levels in women with preeclampsia. Eur *J. Obstet. Gynecol. Reprod. Biol.* 113 (I): 21-25.
[30] Cunningham, F. G., Mac Donald, P. C., Gant, N. F., Leveno, K. J., Gilstrap, L. J., Hankins, G. D. V., Clark, S. L. (2001). Williams *Obstetrics*. 21th edition Connecticut, the McGraw-Hill, p: 567-609.
[31] Sapmaz, E., Bulut, V., Celik, A., Akbulut, H., Ilhan, N., Hanay, F. (2006). Examination of neopterin and TNF-alpha levels in preeclampsia cases. *Turk J Obstet Gynecol*, 3 (II): 83-88.
[32] Saito, S., Shiozaki, A., Nakashima, A., Sakai, M., Sasaki, Y. (2007). The role of the immune system in preeclampsia. *Mol. Aspects Med.* 28 (II): 192-209.
[33] Powe, C. E., Levine, R. J., Karumanchi, S. A. (2011). Preeclampsia, a disease of the maternal endothelium: the role of antiangiogenic

factors and implications for later cardiovascular disease. *Circulation*, 123 (XXIV): 2856-2869.

[34] Hazar, D. (2012). Vascular endothelial growth factor, solubl fms-like tyrosine kinase-1 and endothelin levels in severe preeclampsia and their relationship with each other. Published Ph.D. *Thesis*, Pamukkale University, Denizli.

[35] Romão-Veiga, M., Matias, M. L., Ribeiro, V. R., Nunes, P. R., M Borges, V. T., Peraçoli, J .C., Peraçoli, M. T. S. (2018). Induction of systemic inflammation by hyaluronan and hsp70 in women with pre-eclampsia. *Cytokine*, 105: 23-31.

[36] Myatt, L., Cui, X. (2004). Oxidative stress in the placenta. *Histochem. Cell Biol.* 122 (IV): 369-382.

[37] Zusterzeel, P. L., Rutten, H., Roelofs, H. M., Peters, W. H., Steegers, E. A. (2001). Protein carbonyls in decidua and placenta of pre-eclamtic women as markers for oxidative stress. *Placenta*, 22 (II-III): 213-219.

[38] Von Dadelszen, P., Magee, L. A. (2002). Could an infectious trigger explain the differential maternal response to the shared placental pathology of preeclampsia and normotensive intrauterine growth restriction? *Acta Obstet Gynecol. Scand.* 81 (VII): 642-648.

[39] Sankaralingam, S., Xu, Y., Sawamura, T., Davidge, S. T. (2009). Increased lectin-like oxidized low-density lipoprotein receptor-1 expression in the maternal vasculature of women with preeclampsia: role for peroxynitrite. *Hypertension*, 53 (II): 270-277.

[40] Anton, L., Merrill, D. C., Neves, L. A., Diz, D. I., Corthorn, J., Valdes, G., Stovall, K., Gallagher, P. E., Moorefield, C., Gruver, C., Brosnihan, K. B. (2009). The uterine placental bed Renin-Angiotensin system in normal and preeclamptic pregnancy. *Endocrinology*, 150 (IX): 4316-4325.

In: Preeclampsia
Editor: Torsten Nacht

ISBN: 978-1-53617-116-7
© 2020 Nova Science Publishers, Inc.

Chapter 3

PRE-ECLAMPSIA: PREDICTION, PREVENTION AND TREATMENT

I. V. Lakhno
Kharkin Medical Academy of Postgraduate Education,
Kharkiv, Ukraine

ABSTRACT

The chapter covers the possibilities of the maternal and fetal heart rate variability usage at all stages of management among pre-eclamptic women in a three-stage system.

It has been shown that pre-eclampsia is featured by sympathetic overactivity, vascular spasm, and reduced cardiac output influenced by increased intra-abdominal pressure. The deterioration of uteroplacental circulation was found to decrease the penetration of maternal respiratory sinus arrhythmia through the placental barrier among women with a hypokinetic type of central maternal hemodynamics. These events are captured in the development of maternal multiple organ failure and fetal distress.

The usage of variables of autonomic balance has improved the predictive value of traditional screening of pre-eclampsia by 4.5 times. The application of combined pharmaceutical prophylactics has contributed to the reduction of pre-eclampsia by 8.25 times. The additional screening at 26–28 weeks of pregnancy included maternal heart rate variability parameters which made the selection of contingent for preterm delivery more reasonable.

Keywords: pre-eclampsia, autonomic nervous system, autonomic nervous regulation, heart rate variability, central maternal hemodynamics, fetal distress, systemic inflammatory response syndrome, oxidative stress, antihypertensive drugs.

OBJECTIVES

Pre-eclampsia (PE) is known to be a reason for maternal life-threatening conditions development. PE has a five times higher risk of perinatal mortality. PE is involved in more than 50 thousand maternal deaths annually all over the world [4, 5]. The spread of PE is almost the same in all the regions of the world. It is about 5.0–16.0%. It is known to be unrelated to the level of social and economic development. PE has a negative effect on maternal morbidity from cardiovascular diseases in further lifetime [19, 20, 23].

The initial stage of PE is an ischemic placental syndrome that contributes to the synthesis and release of proinflammatory cytokines and vasoconstrictors into the systemic circulation. An endothelial malfunction and oxidative stress are known to be involved in the PE scenario. These pathological conditions are related to hypercoagulation. An inherited or secondary thrombophilia contributes to the progression of hemostatic disorders. Thus, PE is associated with thrombotic events in the uteroplacental site [1–3, 7, 9].

A number of other pathogenetic mechanisms of PE have already been discovered. The sympathetic overactivity is a reason for increased peripheral vascular resistance, decreased cardiac outflow, and hypoperfusion of a target organ [8, 18, 21]. An increased sympathetic tone is caused by elevated intra-abdominal pressure [24]. Abdominal compartmentalisation is involved in chronic venous insufficiency, hepatic lesion, and systemic inflammatory response syndrome (SIRS). These events contribute to the enhancement for endothelial malfunction and multiple-organ-failure syndrome [22].

Uteroplacental hemodynamics in pre-eclamptic patients is a zone of maximum vascular resistance. This circumstance not only is relevant to placental ischemia but also contributes to fetal deterioration. The disturbed uteroplacental circulation worsens the spreading of maternal autonomic regulation through the placental barrier to the fetus [13]. Therefore, the study of maternal and fetal hemodynamic fluctuations by investigating heart rate variability (HRV) power in all domain regions could be a sensitive biophysical marker of PE. But the pathogenetic role of autonomic disorders is not fully established.

The protocols and algorithms of pre-eclamptic patients' management are not comprehensive and satisfactory. The effective pharmaceutical prevention of PE is a prospect in obstetrical and perinatal medicine. Therefore, the detection of possible 'therapeutic window' for the usage of antiplatelet, vasoactive, and venotonic drugs is still an issue [10, 11, 25]. The maternal and fetal autonomic nervous system monitoring could become a sensitive tool of prediction and diagnosing of and treatment for PE. This systemic approach could contribute to the reduction of PE obstetrical and perinatal complications.

The goal was to improve obstetric and perinatal outcome among pre-eclamptic women by the advancement of a PE prediction, prevention, and treatment system.

MATERIAL AND METHODS

Totally 292 pregnant women were examined. The study was divided into three phases: the selection of the patients, the comparative phase and the cohort prospective study. There were 72 women with a healthy pregnancy in the study. This cohort was divided into three groups according to the gestational age. There were 20 women in the first trimester of pregnancy in Group I. 26 patients at the beginning of the second trimester of pregnancy were enrolled in Group II. There were 26 women at the end of the second or third trimester of pregnancy in Group III. 66 patients with positive biophysical and biochemical markers of PE (pulsatile index in uterine arteries >2,25; PAPP-A <0,69 MoM; β-human chorionic gonadotrophin > 3,0 MoM and α-fetoprotein >2,5 MoM) at the beginning of the second trimester were included in Group IV. This Group was divided into two subgroups. The patients of this Group participated in the prospective cohort study. There were 36 patients who were not received any pharmacological agents for the prevention of PE in Subgroup IV A. 30 pregnant women from IV B Subgroup received low doses of acetylsalicylic acid, diosmin, L-arginine solution, vitamins, and micronutrients containing medication for the prevention of PE. 154 pre-eclamptic women were assigned to main (V) Group. It was divided into subgroups according to the severity of PE: V A – 56 women with mild PE; V B – 53 patients with moderate PE; V C Subgroup – 45 pregnant women with severe PE.

The study protocol was approved by the Bioethics Committee of the Kharkiv Medical Academy of Postgraduate Education. The eligible participants were informed about the study's methodology, its aims, objectives, indications and eventual complications before enrollment. Patients were selected randomly. All the patients who met the inclusion criteria gave written informed consent to participate. The inclusion criteria: diagnosed PE based on the blood pressure higher than 140/90 mm Hg in two separate occasions 6 hours apart, a positive proteinuria test in two midstream urine samples collected 4 hours apart. The exclusion criteria: multiple pregnancies, eclampsia, pre-existing medical disorders like diabetes mellitus, metabolic syndrome, cardiac diseases, renal disease, thyrotoxicosis, and chronic hypertension. If blood pressure was 140 to 159 mmHg systolic and 90 to 109 mmHg the patient was included in mild-moderate PE Group. Severe PE was diagnosed in case of blood pressure was higher 160 mmHg systolic and 110 mmHg diastolic or (and) thrombocytopenia, serum creatinine more than 1.1 mg/L, the elevated blood concentration of liver transaminases to twice normal concentration, pulmonary edema, cerebral or visual disturbances. The patients who had no gestational complications and medical disorders including chronic infections and tobacco smoking were enrolled in the control Group. All patients included in the study were inhabitants of Eastern Ukraine.

All examined pre-eclamptic patients received antihypertensive drugs. The choice of antihypertensive agent was made according to the type of central maternal hemodynamics (CMH) determined by bio-impedance cardiography. It was estimated the values of cardiac index (CI) and total peripheral vascular resistance (TPVR). The hyperkinetic type of CMH was associated with high CI and low TPVR. The pre-eclamptic women with the eukinetic type of CMH had high or normal CI and increased TPVR. And the pre-eclamptic patients with low CI and high TPVR had the hypokinetic type of CMH [17]. The pregnant women with the hyperkinetic type of CMH took carvedilol 6.25-12.5 mg 2 times daily, in case of the eukinetic type – methyldopa 250-500 mg 4 times a day and in cases of the hypokinetic one – methyldopa 500 mg 4 times daily combined with nifedipine 20 mg 2 times daily.

The fetal and maternal HRV parameters were obtained with the fetal noninvasive computer electrocardiographic system "Cardiolab Babycard" (Scientific Research Center "KhAI-Medica", Ukraine). The values of total power (TP) and its spectral compounds, i.e., the very low frequency (VLF), the low frequency (LF), the high frequency (HF) and LF/HF ratio or sympatho-vagal balance, were determined. The temporal characteristics of the fetal HRV: the standard deviation of normal to normal intervals (SDNN), RMSSD, the proportion of the number of pairs of NNs differing by more than 50 ms divided by the total number of NNs (pNN50), the amplitude of mode (the most frequent value of NN interval or the highest column in the histogram) – the number of NN intervals included in the pocket corresponding to the mode measured in percentages (%) (AMo) and the stress index – $SI = AMo(\%)/(2 \times Mo \times Var)$; $Var = NN_{max} - NN_{min}$; (SI) were calculated [13]. CMH types were detected by bioimpedance cardiography on rheographic equipment "Reocom" (Scientific Research Center "KhAI-Medica", Ukraine), Doppler ultrasonography was performed on the ultrasound system "Voluson" (GE Healthcare, USA).

The markers of SIRS, variables of lipid peroxidation and antioxidants, platelet aggregation, coagulation profile, levels of proteins, lipids, macro-, and micronutrients were investigated in blood serum.

The results thus obtained were analyzed with the chi-square test to compare data between groups. For the assessment of the difference between non-parametric variables, the Mann-Whitney test was used. The significance was set at p-value <0.05. For the statistical analysis of the relationship between X and Y, the correlations coefficients were estimated with Spearman's test. SPSS for Windows Release 19,0 (SPSS Inc. Chicago, Illinois), the software was used for statistical analysis. The sensitivity (Se), specificity (Sp), relative risk (RR), and odds ratio (OR) were calculated using MedCalc (MedCalc Software, Mariakerke, Belgium) v.9.6.4.0.

RESULTS AND DISCUSSION

The dominance of the parasympathetic part of the autonomic nervous regulation over the sympathetic one was discovered in a healthy pregnancy (Figure 1). This peculiarity provided gestational regulatory resetting which was supposed to support the growing level of ergo- and trophotropic reactions, and gestational hypervolemia. The growth of the power of a vagal domain region was determined during a paced breathing test in a healthy pregnancy, according to Groups 1, 2, and 3 respectively: 24.2%, 34.4%, and 22.1%. The paradoxical type of reactivity was found in patients of Group 4. The rise of the respiratory sinus arrhythmia related to domain spectral region was only 1.0%. But an unusual increase of an LF power spectrum component by 6.7% was detected. This finding indicates that women with positive biochemical and biophysical markers of PE demonstrate an increased activity of the central sympathetic circuit in the second trimester. The decreased reactivity among pre-eclamptic women was accompanied by a slight increase in the vagal tone domain region power, according to Subgroups 5 A, 5 B, and 5 C, respectively: 5.7%, 7.3%, and 15.6%. The reduction in the parasympathetic tone power was observed among women with PE in addition to the sympathetic overactivity. Therefore, the paced breathing testing has confirmed that overactivity of the sympathetic tone was associated with a certain decrease in the parasympathetic part of the PE autonomic nervous regulation.

The hemodynamic effect found in the position of a pregnant woman lying on her right side was associated with an increased sympathetic tone and captured the circulatory response to the compression of the aorta and inferior cava vein. This mechanism of hemodynamic regulation should compensate for decreased venous return as a result of aortic compression by increasing sympathetic effects on the vascular tone. The abdominal vessels' compression by the pregnant uterus was the same among women of Group 2 and Group 4, but at the same time, the sympatho-vagal balance was almost two times higher among Group 4 patients. Therefore, the additional contribution to the compression of large vessels may have been caused by increased intraabdominal pressure, which was the cause for the activation of the maternal sympathetic centres. Thus, the important event in the development of PE was an excessive growth of the intra-abdominal pressure.

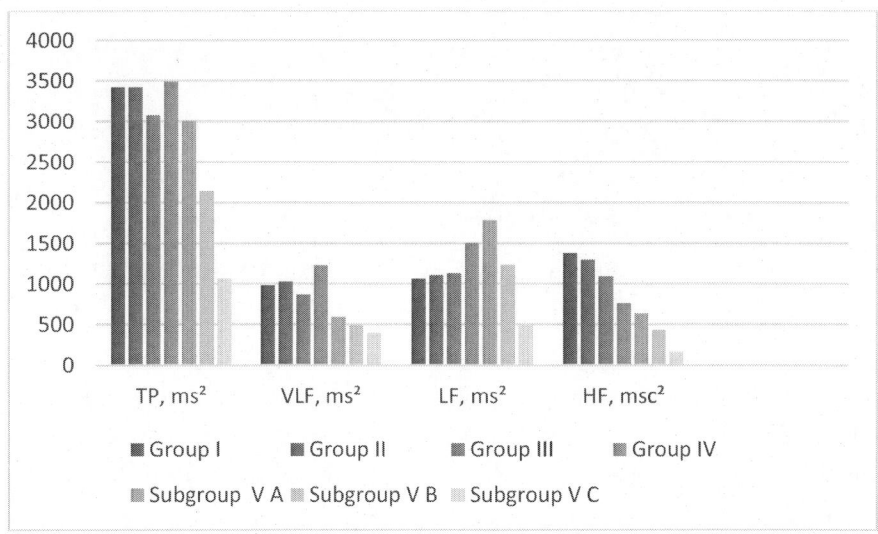

Figure 1. A sympatho-vagal balance in the study population.

The orthostatic position caused a decrease in the total power of HRV and the high-frequency domain region. The sympathetic overactivity could not have the ability to improve the disturbed hemodynamics among pre-eclamptic women and worsened the arterial and venous blood flow.

The performed investigation has led us to the assumption that PE developed on the background of the elevated CI. The presence of the hyperkinetic type of CMH was found in the majority of patients with mild or moderate PE. The hypervolemia and normal or slightly elevated TPVR persisted among this contingent of the study population.

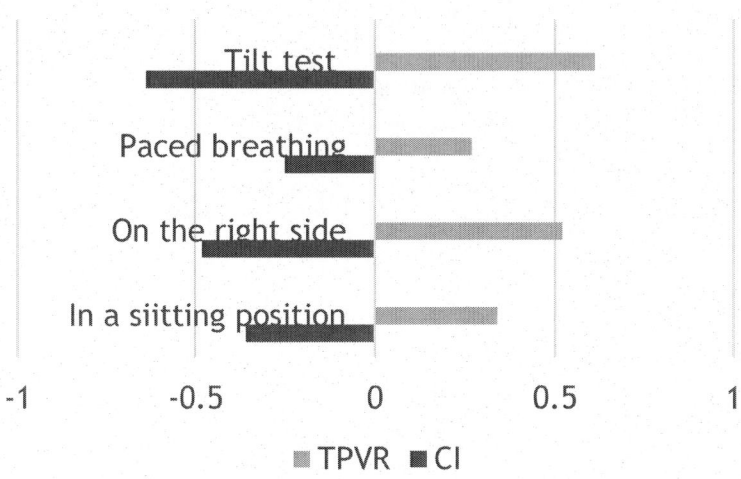

Figure 2. The correlation between TPVR, CI, and sympatho-vagal balance.

The increased vascular permeability, hypovolemia, and low CI have been characterised by the hypokinetic type of CMH in the case of the severity progression of PE. The sympathetic overactivity could be considered as a compensatory response supported by the perfusion of an end organ in mild and moderate PE. The correlation between the sympatho-vagal balance and CI ($r_s = -0.64$; $p < 0.05$), sympatho-vagal balance and TPVR ($r_s = 0.61$; $p < 0.05$) was found in the tilt test (Figure 2).

The maximal growth of a sympatho-vagal balance was related to the suppression of the respiratory sinus arrhythmia, hypokinetic type of CMH in patients with severe PE. There were signs of hemodynamics centralisation and hypoperfusion of an end organ in these women. PE was featured by the destruction of the basic gestational vagal-dependent mechanism of fluid retention and vasodilation in a general case.

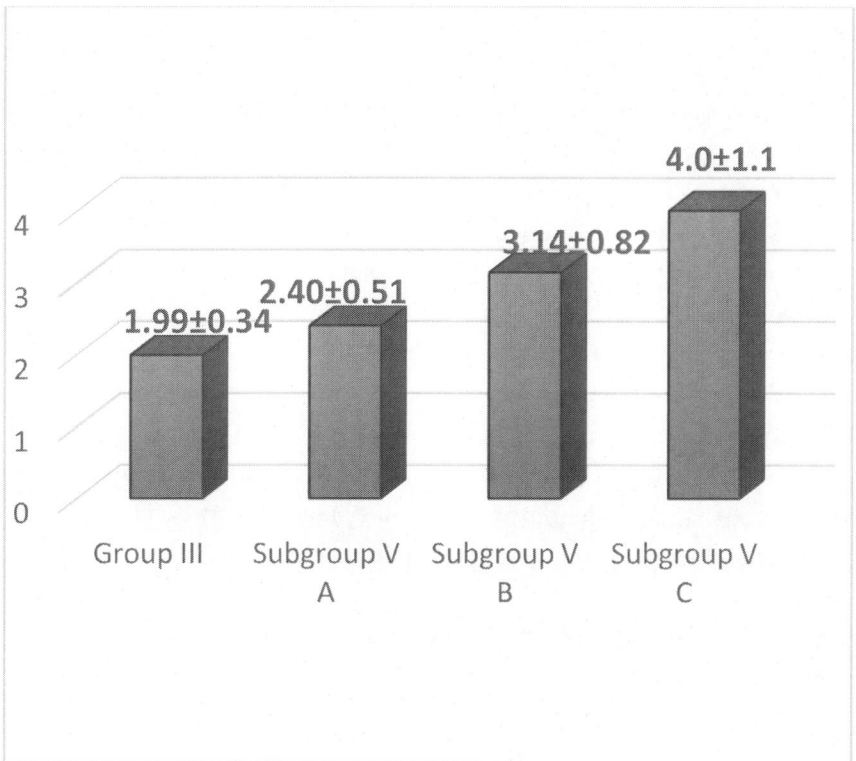

Figure 3. Fetal sympatho-vagal balance in PE.

The increased fetal vagal tone by the end of gestation among healthy pregnancy group women can be considered to be a sign of fetal maturity. Depending on the progredient severity of PE, there were suppression of fetal autonomic tone, sympathetic overactivity, and low vagal tone. Thus, an increased sympathetic tone played a significant role in the development of fetal distress in PE.

The supression of fetal autonomic nervous regulation, combined with sympathetic overactivity, fetal cardiac conduction abnormalties, and decreased uteroplacental hemodynamics, were found in PE [13, 14].

Non-invasive fetal ECG was a convenient and informative method of antenatal fetal monitoring. The appearance of decelerations as a reaction to the intrauterine fetal motile activity suggests fetal distress. An additional study of the QT interval and the T/QRS ratio can confirm or refute this diagnosis. Thus, the use of non-invasive fetal ECG has made it possible to improve the accuracy of the fetal distress diagnosis [14].

The performed investigations have made it possible to determine the effect of the maternal autonomic nervous regulation on fetal hemodynamics. The relationship between maternal respiratory sinus arrhythmia and umbilical venous circulation was supported by revealed correlation (rs = 0.62; p < 0.05). The maternal respiratory sinus arrhythmia could be one of the drivers of blood flow in the umbilical vein at a healthy pregnancy. The lack of parasympathetic regulation in pre-eclamptic women and deterioration of placental hemodynamics had a decreased impact on umbilical circulation. This contributed to the pulsatile pattern of blood flow in the umbilical vein and the development of fetal distress. Thus, hemodynamic isolation of the fetus was an important pathogenetic event of fetal distress in women suffering from PE [13, 15].

Table 1. The variables of correlation between proinflammatory cytokines, C- reactive protein (C-RP), maternal and fetal HRV in PE

HRV variables	IL-1β	IL-6	TNF-α	C-RP
Maternal TP	$r_s = -0.50$	$r_s = -0.54$	$r_s = -0.46$	$r_s = -0.41$
Maternal VLF	$r_s = -0.48$	$r_s = -0.45$	$r_s = -0.54$	$r_s = 0.42$
Maternal LF	$r_s = 0.68$	$r_s = 0.61$	$r_s = 0.55$	$r_s = 0.50$
Maternal HF	$r_s = -0.46$	$r_s = -0.60$	$r_s = -0.58$	$r_s = -0.56$
Fetal TP	$r_s = -0.48$	$r_s = -0.44$	$r_s = -0.40$	$r_s = -0.45$
Fetal VLF	$r_s = -0.36$	$r_s = -0.38$	$r_s = -0.32$	$r_s = -0.44$
Fetal LF	$r_s = 0.43$	$r_s = 0.44$	$r_s = 0.41$	$r_s = 0.38$
Fetal HF	$r_s = -0.48$	$r_s = -0.55$	$r_s = -0.44$	$r_s = -0.46$

'Physiological' inflammation was a satellite of pregnancy starting from the first trimester. The process of trophoblast invasion initiated a slight increase in concentrations of proinflammatory cytokines and C-reactive protein. The SIRS was found in women with PE in the third trimester of pregnancy. The mediators of chronic inflammation influenced the maternal autonomic nervous regulation and participated in the development of fetal distress (Table 1). Perhaps, the sympathetic part of the autonomic nervous system had an immunomodulating effect associated with increased production of pro-inflammatory cytokines, whereas the parasympathetic part had a reverse relation to pro-inflammatory mediators [12, 16].

The activation of blood coagulation, an increased vascular-platelet component of hemostasis, and the suppression of the anticoagulant system were found in patients with PE. Hypercoagulation was stimulated by the pro-inflammatory mediators. The thrombophilia was featured by a hypocoagulation and an impaired platelet function in women with severe PE. This caused the low platelet count and decreased platelet aggregation. The sympathetic division of the autonomic nervous system was found to contribute to hypercoagulation, but the parasympathetic one had a stimulating effect on the endogenous anticoagulant system [6].

The stimulating impact of the adrenergic substances on the variables of platelet aggregation captured the progredient endothelial malfunction. The atherogenic dyslipidemia was detected in pre-eclamptic women. Therefore, the functional properties of the endothelium and blood cells depended on the state of lipid metabolism, the system of lipid peroxidation and antioxidants [15, 16].

Oxidative stress had a negative influence on the metabolism of micronutrients. Pre-eclamptic women had fluid and electrolyte imbalance, a decrease in the number of anti-inflammatory and membrane-protecting nutrients: calcium, magnesium, zinc, and, on the other hand, an increase in the level of proinflammatory and prooxidant nutrient—copper [12, 21, 25].

Thus, PE developed under the influence of sympathetic overactivity, which contributed to the development of thrombophilia, dyslipidemia, oxidative stress, endothelial dysfunction, and imbalance of macro- and micronutrients. The maternal autonomic imbalance could be of great importance in the pathogenesis of PE, both with early and late onset. The enhanced sympathetic tone contributed to the growth of the intra-abdominal pressure. The increased power of the sympathetic division of the maternal autonomic nervous regulation had a reflexion on fetal hemodynamics deterioration and participated in the pathogenesis of fetal distress [13, 15].

It was found during the prospective observation that OR of a positive result for PE in Subgroup 4 A was 16.5. The additional use of sympatho-vagal balance variables in maternal position on the right side and in the active orthostatic test increased the predictive value of screening of PE with an increase of OR up to 74.4. The changes in the autonomous balance increased the predictive value of the biophysical and biochemical tests by 4.5 times. The Se and Sp for the proposed protocol of screening were 90.3% and 84.8%, respectively.

The proposed pharmaceutical intervention for the prevention of PE used in women of Subgroup 4 B confirmed its significant clinical efficacy. This conclusion was supported by a decrease in the OR by 8.25 times. The performed intervention contributed not only to the reduction of the rate of PE in women at risk but also to the postponement of its manifestation. There were no cases of early-onset PE in Subgroup 4 B. We have found that the proposed pharmaceutical prevention of PE can improve the autonomic nervous regulation of the mother and fetus. The calculation of RR determined that the use of the suggested pharmaceutical intervention decreased the RR of preterm birth by 4.2 times, poor progress of labour—by 1.7, postpartum haemorrhages—by 3.0, cesarean delivery—by 3.0, hypogalactia—by 1.9, fetal distress—by 2.5, fetal growth restriction—by 3.3, prenatal encephalopathy—by 1.9, respiratory distress—by 2.3, jaundice—by 2.1, and perinatal infection—by 2.5.

The variables of CI and TPVR did not have any significant dynamics in the process of treatment of pre-eclamptic women. The obtained data indicate that the initial type of CMH mostly persisted in patients suffering from PE who have used antihypertensive drugs [17]. Since some decrease of cardiac index values was found in pre-eclamptic women in all subgroups, the antihypertensive drugs were not able to reestablish the adaptive mechanisms of the maternal cardiovascular system. Thus, antihypertensive therapy for PE was aimed at prevention of intracranial hemorrhage rather than provision of the optimal regimen of the CMH.

The positive dynamics of the separate instrumental and laboratory parameters of pre-eclamptic patients was observed in the postpartum period. The variables of blood pressure were found to become safer. The decrease in the intra-abdominal pressure could have been contributed to the improved maternal circulation. However, the persisted increased sympathetic tone observed on the third day of puerperium was caused by the increased influence of the central sympathetic circuit. It contributed to the persistence of hypovolemia and peripheral vasoconstriction. Therefore, a definite period of taking antihypertensive drugs is necessary for rehabilitation of patients with severe PE.

CONCLUSION

The possible way to improve the maternal and perinatal outcomes is following the three-step system of management of women at risk of PE. The first step is an early beginning of pharmaceutical intervention for the prevention of PE in women with internal diseases or complicated obstetrical anamnesis. The patients with diseases associated with an increased level of cytokines and systemic vasculopathy should be under a special care. The screening for biochemical and biophysical markers of PE at the end of the first or at the beginning of the second trimester of pregnancy is performed as a second step. There is a study of sympatho-vagal balance in the sitting position, lying on the right side, and the active orthostatic test, the investigation of the pulsatile index in the uterine arteries, the blood serum concentrations of pregnancy-associated plasma protein A, β-human chorionic gonadotrophin and α-fetoprotein among these markers. In the case of an increased risk of PE, pharmaceutical intervention is recommended before 16 weeks of gestation. The third step is a remedy for early diagnosis of PE at the end of the second trimester or the beginning of the third trimester. The main task is to determine the target population of women that require hospitalisation and preterm delivery. Since there is still no effective treatment for PE, the emphasis should be made on its prevention and timely pregnancy termination.

REFERENCES

[1] Aguilar A. Pre-eclampsia: sFLT1 inhibits NO signalling//*Nat Rev Nephrol.* – 2016. – Vol. 12, No 8. – P. 442.

[2] Ali S. M., Khalil R. A. Genetic, immune and vasoactive factors in the vascular dysfunction associated with hypertension in pregnancy//*Expert Opin Ther Targets.* – 2015. – Vol. 19, No 11. – P. 1495–1515.

[3] Ann-Charlotte I. Inflammatory mechanisms in preeclampsia//*Pregnancy Hypertens.* – 2013. – Vol. 3, No 2. – P. 58.

[4] Berhan Y. No Hypertensive disorder of pregnancy; no preeclampsia-eclampsia; no gestational hypertension; no hellp syndrome. Vascular disorder of pregnancy speaks for all//*Ethiop J Health Sci.* – 2016. – Vol. 26, No 2. – P. 177–186.

[5] Burgess A., Founds S. Cardiovascular implications of preeclampsia//*MCN Am J Matern Child Nurs.* – 2016. – Vol. 41, No 1. – P. 8–15.

[6] Crotty T. P. The balance between the pro-inflammatory effect of plasma noradrenaline and the anti-inflammatory effect of neuronal noradrenaline determines the peripheral effects of noradrenaline//*Med Hypotheses.* – 2015. – Vol. 85, No 5. – P. 517–529.

[7] Das U. N. Cytokines, angiogenic, and antiangiogenic factors and bioactive lipids in preeclampsia//*Nutrition.* – 2015. – Vol. 31, No 9. – P. 1083–1095.

[8] 8, Dennis A. T. Management of pre-eclampsia: issues for anaesthetists//*Anaesthesia.* – 2012. – Vol. 67, No 9. – P. 1009–1020.

[9] Eggers A. E. A suggestion about the cause of inflammation in acute atherosis complicating poor placentation in preeclampsia//Med Hypotheses. –2015. – Vol. 85, No 6. – P. 718–719.
[10] Friedman A. M., Cleary K. L. Prediction and prevention of ischemic placental disease//*Semin Perinatol.* – 2014. – Vol. 38, No 3. – P. 177–182.
[11] Herrera J. A. Primary prevention of preeclampsia: myth or reality?//*Colomb Med (Cali).* – 2015. – Vol. 46, No 4. – P. 154–155.
[12] Huston M., Tracey K. J. The pulse of inflammation: heart rate variability, the cholinergic anti-inflammatory pathway and implications for therapy//*J Int Med.* – 2011. – Vol. 269, No 1. – P. 45–53.
[13] Lakhno I. Autonomic response determines fetal and maternal interaction in pre-eclampsia/In book: *Neurological Perspectives of Autonomic Dysfunctions,* Chapter: Chapter 3, Publisher: Nova Science Publishers (New York), 2016. – Editors: Peter Freeman. – P. 85–101.
[14] Lakhno I. Fetal non-invasive electrocardiography contributes to better diagnostics of fetal distress: a cross-sectional study among patients with pre-eclampsia//*Ann. Acad. Med. Singapore.* – 2015. – Vol. 44, No 11. – P. 519–523.
[15] Lakhno I. Maternal respiratory sinus arrhythmia captures the severity of pre-eclampsia//*Archives of Perinatal Medicine.* – 2016. – Vol. 22, No 2. – P. 14–17.
[16] Lakhno I. The role of maternal inflammation in fetal and maternal autonomic dysfunction in preeclamptic patients//*Archives of Perinatal Medicine.* – 2015. – Vol. 21, No 1. – P. 22–25.
[17] Lakhno I. V. Antihypertensive drugs impact on the regulation of maternal and fetal cardiac activity in pregnant women with preeclampsia//*The New Armenian Medical Journal.* – 2015. – Vol. 9, No 1. – P. 58–62.
[18] Maeda K. Electroencephalographic studies of eclampsia and pre-eclampsia//*J Obstet Gynaecol Res.* – 2016. – Vol. 42, No 1. – P. 11–20.

[19] Murphy M. S., Smith G. N. Pre-eclampsia and cardiovascular disease risk assessment in women//*Am J Perinatol.* – 2016. – Vol. 33, No 8. – P. 723–731.
[20] Phillips C., Boyd M. Assessment, management, and health implications of early-onset preeclampsia//*Nurs Womens Health.* – 2016. –Vol. 20, No 4. – P. 400–414.
[21] Polonia J. Preeclampsia: a fascinating syndrome due not only to oxidative stress//*Rev Port Cardiol.* –2016. – Vol. 35, No 9. – P. 477–478.
[22] Redman C. W., Staff A. C. Preeclampsia, biomarkers, syncytiotrophoblast stress, and placental capacity//*Am J Obstet Gynecol.* – 2015. – Vol. 213, No 4 (Suppl). – S. 9. e1, S 9–11.
[23] Rosser M. L., Katz N. T. Preeclampsia: an obstetrician's perspective//Adv Chronic Kidney Dis. – 2013. – Vol. 20, No 3. – P. 287–296.
[24] Sugerman H. J. Hypothesis: preeclampsia is a venous disease secondary to an increased intra-abdominal pressure//*Med Hypotheses.* – 2011. – Vol. 77, No 5. – P. 841–849.
[25] Young B. C., Karumanchi S. A. Toward a better diagnosis for preeclampsia//*Clin Chem.* – 2016. – Vol. 62, No 7. – P. 913–915.

In: Preeclampsia
Editor: Torsten Nacht

ISBN: 978-1-53617-116-7
© 2020 Nova Science Publishers, Inc.

Chapter 4

PRE-ECLAMPSIA MANAGEMENT PROBLEMS TODAY

Alena I. Baranouskaya[*]
Department of Obstetrics and Gynecology Belarusian State Medical University Minsk, Belarus

ABSTRACT

This review includes sources of literature with a purpose of the systematization of modern information on pathogenesis, management and the long-term consequences of pre-eclampsia. There is scientific evidence of the role of soluble Fms-like tyrosine kinase-1and angiogenic growth factors in the pathogenesis of preeclampsia. However, modern science does not exactly know the etiology of preeclampsia. Therefore, the only way ofterminating preeclampsia is giving a childbirth. Successful management of preeclampsia involves coherent, correct steps. In a patient with arterial hypertension, it is necessary to conduct a differential diagnosis, assess the severity of preeclampsia and confirm the condition of the fetus. Criteria for the diagnosis of preeclampsia are known, but problems with the treatment of this pathology still remains. Delivery is necessary for women with severe or progressive preeclampsia. In all

---

[*] Corresponding Author Email: elena_baranovska@mail.ru.

countries, it is recommended to use magnesium sulphate for the prevention and treatment of eclampsia and to use corticosteroids for prevention neonatal complications in case of premature pregnancy. The long-term consequences of preeclampsia are cardiovascular diseases and the resulting death.

Keywords: pre-eclampsia, hypertension, pregnancy, delivery, magnesium sulphate

INTRODUCTION

Pre-eclampsia is a serious complication of pregnancy, the essence of which lies in multiorgan dysfunction in women with disadaptation to the needs of the fetoplacental system. The word "*pre-eclampsia*" includes two parts: "*pre-*" in the meaning of "*before*" and "*eclampsia*" from the Greek "*eklampo*," which is translated as "*flare up,*" "*ignite.*" The term preeclampsia exactly refers to the pathophysiological process that precedes the acute critical state - eclampsia, so this term has been used in the world for more than 100 years (Ehrenfest 1920, 214).

Preeclampsia refers to hypertensive disorders in pregnant women, since high blood pressure is the most noticeable and most significant symptom of preeclampsia with a large variety of other symptoms. Hypertensive disorders in pregnant women include, along with preeclampsia, also chronic hypertension and gestational hypertension without significant proteinuria. The frequency of general cases preeclampsia is without significant changes, but share of severe cases of preeclampsia is increasing. A population study in the United States from 1980 to 2010 showed a prevalence of preeclampsia of 3.4% in 1980 and 3.8% in 2010. At the same time, the number of mild pre-eclampsia decreased from 3.1% to 2.5%, while the number of severe pre-eclampsia increased from 0.3% to 1.4%. The authors believe that these changes are due to the transition from mild to severe pre-eclampsia (Ananth et al. 2013). The frequency of pre-eclampsia in Australia for the period 2000-2008 was 3.3% with a decreasing trend. However, the incidence of eclampsia increased significantly from 2.3% in 2000 to 4.2% in 2008 and is 8.6 per 10,000 births. The contribution of pre-eclampsia to early maternal mortality (42 days after delivery) is 17% (Thornton et al. 2013, 476.e1).

Preeclampsia significantly affects maternal and neonatal mortality and morbidity (Langenveld et al. 2011, 540.e4; Nathan et al. 2018, 186). WHO estimates that the world's most common causes of maternal death are bleeding 27.1% (19.9–36.2) and hypertension (14.0%, 11.1–17.4) (Say et al. 2014, e327). Preeclampsia in the structure of maternal mortality varies from country to country and depends on the measures taken to prevent and manage preeclampsia. A successful reduction in maternal death from pre-eclampsia and eclampsia has been achieved in the UK. In the UK in 2006–2008, there were 19 dead, in 2009–2011 already 10, and in the following 2012–2014 less than one woman died from pre-eclampsia and eclampsia. These favorable results are achieved thanks to good antenatal care, the introduction of the UK National Health Service guidelines (Shennan et al. 2017, 582).

DEFINITIONS

Hypertensive disorders in pregnant women include chronic hypertension, gestational hypertension, pre-eclampsia (and eclampsia), as well as pre-eclampsia, which is superimposed on chronic hypertension (Task Force on Hypertension in Pregnancy 2013, 1123; Lowe et al. 2015, 11).

Chronic hypertension is characterized by systolic blood pressure (SBP)> 140 mmHg, diastolic blood pressure (DBP)> 90 mmHg, confirmed by at least two measurements with an interval of at least four hours outside of pregnancy, childbirth and the postpartum period or during first half of pregnancy (up to 20 weeks).

Gestational hypertension - increased blood pressure (SBP > 140 mmHg, DBP> 90 mmHg), which occurred for the first time after 20 weeks of pregnancy, without significant proteinuria, namely, without proteinuria or with a protein concentration in the urine less than 0.3 g in daily portion of urine. Gestational hypertension can only be diagnosed during pregnancy. According to the International Society for the Study of Hypertension in Pregnancy (ISSHP), for gestational hypertension, blood pressure returns to normal within 12 weeks after delivery.

If blood pressure rises after 20 weeks of pregnancy or during childbirth and in the postpartum period, while proteinuria > 0.3 g of protein per daily urine, then these are signs of pre-eclampsia. The definition of "Pre-eclampsia" can be formulated as follows. *Pre-eclampsia* is a syndrome of polyorgan dysfunction that occurs during pregnancy and is caused by the failure of the mother's adaptation systems to meet the needs of the developing fetus.

Often, pre-eclampsia occurs in previously existing chronic hypertension. In this case, high blood pressure existed before pregnancy and continues to exist throughout pregnancy, to this, after 20 weeks of pregnancy, proteinuria and other signs of polyorgan dysfunction appear.

Signs of eclampsia are convulsions and/or coma with previous signs of preeclampsia.

PATHOGENESIS

Until recently, it was known that endothelial damage, vasoconstriction, perfusion disturbance, ischemia and organ hypoxia are the main factors of multiorgan dysfunction in preeclampsia. This mechanism is explained by the pathological invasion of cytotrophoblast into the spiral arteries of the uterus and the subsequent angiogenic imbalance (Magee et al. 2014, 110).

Nowadays, the world scientific community has recognized that the cause of endothelial dysfunction, which forms the basis of the pre-eclampsia pathogenesis, is precisely the angiogenic imbalance. Endothelial damage is associated with exposure to soluble Fms-like tyrosine kinase-1 (sFlt-1), which is a soluble receptor for vascular endothelial growth factor-1 (sVEGFR1). sFlt-1 is a strong circulating antagonist of both vascular endothelial growth factor (VEGF) a nd placental growth factor (PlGF) which is necessary for neoangiogenesis and the formation of the placental complex. Excess of sFlt-1 causes endothelial damage and vasoconstriction. For PlGF, this was proven in a multicentre trialin 11 maternity units in the UK involving 1023 women suspected of preeclampsia in 2016–2017 (Duhig et al. 2019, 1813). The sFlt-1/PlGF ratio is referred to as a negative prognostic criteria for preeclampsia (Zeisler et al. 2016,19). However, both sFlt-1 and PlGF did not show their usefulness for first trimester screening as predictors of pre-eclampsia (Schneuer et al. 2013, 218), they also cannot be used to differentiate hypertensive disorders in pregnant women (SOMANZ 2014, 7).

DIAGNOSIS

The pathophysiological process of pre-eclampsia begins at a very early gestational period, but clinical signs appear after 20 weeks of gestation. Rarely, pre-eclampsia manifests for the first time in childbirth or the postpartum period. Preeclampsia is a multisystem syndrome, including hypertension and signs of dysfunction of one or more systems of vital organs of the mother and/or fetus. Increased blood pressure is one of the earliest, visible, and easily detectable symptoms. The appearance and intensity of other symptoms of preeclampsia depend on the damaged organ (kidney, liver, brain, placenta) and system (vascular, hemocoagulation).

There are two degrees of severity of pre-eclampsia - middle and severe. This separation of pre-eclampsia helps the doctor in choosing a strategy. With a middle degree of pre-eclampsia on the term of less than 37 weeks of gestation, pregnancy can be continued to the full term, provided adequate treatment, controlled hypertension, stable condition of the mother and fetus. Severe preeclampsia is an indication for termination of pregnancy.

The criteria for the diagnosis of pre-eclampsia include a combination of hypertension with any signs of dysfunction of one or more other organ systems and/or the fetus: renal, hematological, hepatic, neurological, pulmonary, placental. Disorders of the placenta, used as criteria for the diagnosis of pre-eclampsia, are fetal growth retardation, abnormal fetal heart rhythm, oligohydramnion, absence or reverse diastolic blood flow according to Doppler, premature placental abruption. Diastolic blood pressure is more significant for clinical evaluation and diagnosis. If systolic and diastolic blood pressure are in different categories, the severity of hypertension is assessed according to the highest figure.

Differential diagnosis of preeclampsia should be carried out with chronic hypertension, gestational hypertension. The main differences are in the timing of detection of arterial hypertension and the presence of polysystem dysfunction (table).

Table. Differential diagnosis of hypertensive disorders in pregnant women

Hypertensive disorders	Time to detect hypertension				System dysfunction
	before pregnancy	<20 weeks of gestation	>20 weeks of gestation	after postpartum	
chronic hypertension	Yes	Yes	Yes	Yes	No
gestational hypertension	No	No	Yes	No	No
pre-eclampsia	No	No	Yes	No	Yes
pre-eclampsia superimposed on chronic hypertension	Yes	Yes	Yes	Yes	Yes

The following clinical and instrumental methods of research are used for the differential diagnosis of pre-eclampsia, assessment of its dynamics, control over the effectiveness of treatment:

- blood pressure monitoring,
- measurement of proteinuria,
- measurement of blood biochemical parameters to assess the function of the liver and kidneys (AlAT, AsAT, alkaline phosphatase, bilirubin, creatinine),

- hemostasiogram,
- assessment of hemoconcentration (increased hemoglobin, hematocrit) and platelet count in the blood,
- fundus examination to assess the condition of the retina and blood vessels,
- assessment of neurological status.

Diagnosis of placental disorders includes:

- dopplerometry of the placenta and fetus,
- cardiotocography,
- ultrasound for the diagnosis of growth retardation and condition of the placenta.

Edemas do not have independent diagnostic value. Exceptions are generalized or rapidly progressive edema.

It is important to differentiate the severity of pre-eclampsia. Signs of severe pre-eclampsia include significant hypertension with multiple organ dysfunction with a combination of criteria:

- systolic blood pressure ≥ 160 mm Hg or diastolic blood pressure ≥ 110 mm Hg in two dimensions after 4 hours or more with patient's bed rest
- and/or
- presence of signs of organ dysfunction, biochemical and hematological changes: thrombocytopenia, liver dysfunction, progressive renal failure, pulmonary edema, brain or visual disorders.

There is a proposal to use both the PlGF and sFlt-1 indicators to diagnose preeclampsia (Black and da Silva Costa 2018, 9-26)and it has economic benefits (Figueira et al. 2018, 33).

PRE-ECLAMPSIA MANAGEMENT

Management of Pregnancy with Pre-Eclampsia

Genesis of preeclampsia is associated with the maladaptation of a pregnant woman to the needs of the fetus, therefore it is impossible to get rid of preeclampsia during pregnancy. However, it is possible to stabilize the condition of a pregnant woman with adequate treatment. Without treatment, preeclampsia progresses and the intensity of progress is difficult to predict.

The objectives pursued in the management of pre-eclampsia are, firstly, the preservation of the mother's health and life, secondly, the birth of a live, full-term newborn who does not need intensive care. It is important to make the right decision regarding gestational age for childbirth, evaluate the condition of the cervix for induction of labor or indications for cesarean section, and at the same time conduct preeclampsia therapy.

In especial cases, emergency labor is necessary to save the mother's life, regardless of the gestational age of the fetus. The choice of a general strategy for the management of pre-eclampsia depends on its severity, gestational age, the condition of the fetus. Resistant to treatment severe pre-eclampsiais an indication for childbirth in the interests of the mother. With middle preeclampsia and a compensated fetal condition with adequate therapy, it is best to continue the pregnancy up to 37 weeks so that the fetus becomes mature.

As soon as pre-eclampsia was diagnosed, this is the reason of the patient's hospitalization. Patients with preeclampsia should be monitored daily for blood pressure, proteinuria, and fetal heart rhythm. Ultrasound with doppler, daily fetal movement count and, if necessary, a biophysical profile should also be performed to assess the condition of the fetus. The patient's stay in the hospital allows monitoring blood pressure using antihypertensive drugs, if necessary,prescribing sedatives, titrating magnesium sulfate, examining the uteroplacental blood flow, performing laboratory tests. Laboratory control includes measurement of proteinuria, hematocrit, platelets, transaminases, fibrinogen, D-dimers. Daily observation makes it possible to assess the signs of predictors of eclampsia, such as persistent headache, visual disturbances, the rapid spread of edema. Pregnancy can continue under the condition of controlled stable blood pressure, the absence of significant proteinuria and other adverse symptoms in the mother, the normal state of the fetus. Daily home care with the participation of medical staff is possible in countries where outpatient care is organized for pregnant women with mild pre-eclampsia with mild hypertension. In this case, the patient should be well instructed with regard to home mode, measurement of proteinuria and blood pressure, evaluation of fetal movements and self-perception. When signs of progress of pre-eclampsia appear, hospitalization is needed. The best is the continuation of pregnancy up to 37 weeks, after which a favorable cervix is an indication for induction of labor. Such tactics are justified to prevent the progress of preeclampsia, reduce the risk of maternal death and increase fetal survival.

The risk of maternal and neonatal mortality increases significantly if middlepre-eclampsia becomes severe, fetal condition worsens, pregnancy complications appear, such as placental abruption. The patient should be transferred to a tertiary or quaternary perinatal center for labor at a gestational age of less than 36 weeks for optimal perinatal care. There is a general agreement on the need for childbirth, when gestational age is 34 weeks in pregnant women with severe pre-eclampsia. At the same time, there are different points of view regarding childbirth at an age of less than 34 weeks with severe pre-eclampsia, but in general, individual management is required. For the prevention of seizures in pregnant women, parenteral magnesium sulfate should be prescribed. There is a reason to prescribe corticosteroids to achieve maturity of the lungs of the fetus at a period of 28-34 weeks. For this purpose, pregnancy should be continued for at least 48 hours, provided that the mother and fetus are in well-being stable condition. This measure reduces the stay of the newborn in the intensive care unit.

Improvement of the perinatal outcome is possible with expectant management with a patient's good response to therapy and an increase in gestation age. The expected management of severe pre-eclampsia is justified when the gestation period is less than 34 weeks, and is possible only with strict control and good patient response to treatment only in a tertiary care centre (Sibai 2011, 193). For expectant management of severe pre-eclampsia before 34 weeks, the patient is admitted to the intensive care unit, continuous administration of magnesium sulfate is prescribed to prevent seizures, antihypertensive drugs to achieve a diastolic pressure no higher than 110 mm Hg. Assessment of the mother's condition includes monitoring of blood pressure, heart rate, diuresis, neurological status, monitoring of the level of platelets and liver enzymes. At the same time assess the condition of the fetus - heart rate monitoring, ultrasonography. If there is no response to therapy or there are any signs of maternal or fetal impairment, this is an indication for delivery within 24 hours. If a good response to treatment is given, the pregnancy continues, but the patient should remain in the tertiary care centre, because there are no reliable predictors for predicting pre-eclampsia.

Childbirth

Years of experience shows that only childbirth relieves preeclampsia and prevents eclampsia in a woman. Therefore, in full-term pregnancy with preeclampsia, the objective is to correctly evaluate either there are indications for cesarean section or if the cervix is favorable for induction of labor. At the same time, it is necessary to maintain a stable good condition of the mother and to prevent eclampsia.

If pre-eclampsia is severe and pregnancy is preterm the objective is more difficult. In the case of a premature pregnancy, there is a "conflict of interests" between the mother and the fetus: full gestational age at birth is best for the fetus, but to preserve the health and life of the mother in a serious or progressive deteriorating condition, immediate delivery is required regardless of gestational age (Magee et al. 2014, 111).Cochrane review confirms high risk of neonatal adverse conditions in severe pre-eclampsia with intervention up to week 34 (Churchill et al. 2018, 42).

Recommendations for childbirth in women with preeclampsia and premature pregnancy are listed in Clinical Practice Guidelines (CPGs) of the American College of Obstetrics and Gynecology, the Society of Obstetricians and the Gynaecologists of Canada, National Institute of Health and Care Excellence (UK). In accordance with these CPGs at a gestational age of up to 24 weeks, the patient should be informed in advance about the upcoming birth and notified of the high risk of adverse perinatal outcome. After 24-34 weeks with a stable condition of the mother, pregnancy should be managed expectantly. For women with severe pre-eclampsia, immediate delivery is recommended, even at less than 34 weeks.

In favor of expectant management of severe pre-eclampsia, it should be taken into account that before 34 weeks an increase in gestational age even by 1-2 weeks significantly improves neonatal outcome (ACOG 2017, e188). There is a report oninfants who were born at 22 to 24 weeks of gestation at 11 centers that participated in the National Institute of Child Health and Human Development Neonatal Research Network. Only 1% of 234 born survived without neurological disorders at the gestational age of 22 weeks, at 23 weeks 13% of 450 newborns and at 24 weeks 32% of 664 newborns in the period of 2008-2011 (Younge et al. 2017, 623). A similar study from 2006-2011 at 24 hospitals shows that survival without moderate or severe impairment of those born at the gestational age of 22 weeks is not, at 23 weeks - 14.2%, at 24 weeks -30.5%, 25 weeks - 46.5%, at 26 weeks - 59.8% (Rysavy et al. 2015, 1807).

Indicators for childbirth in women with preeclampsia are gestational age of 37 weeks or more, severe treatment-resistant preeclampsia for any gestational age, fetal disorders. With favorable cervix and the absence of severe maternal and fetal disorders induction of labor is an indication (Coviello et al. 2019, 100.e4). During vaginal delivery, continuous monitoring of fetal heartbeats and uterine activity, blood pressure control, and drug anesthesia are required. In the case of unripe cervix, very early preterm labor, a decision should be made on a cesarean section.

Blood pressure monitoring, laboratory monitoring should be continued for at least 24 hours after delivery, along with the appointment of antihypertensive drugs and magnesium sulfate. Women with severe preeclampsia need long-term treatment and follow-up after delivery.

Antihypertensive Drugs

Systolic blood pressure ≥ 140 mmHg. and/or diastolic blood pressure ≥ 90 mm Hg. are the criterias for hypertension diagnosis. The same criterias are applicable to preeclampsia diagnosis. However, after 20 weeks of gestation, specific hemodynamic occur, therefore baseline blood pressure values for starting therapy and target blood pressure values may be individual and change with gestational age. The Society of Obstetric Medicine of Australia and New Zealand considers the treatment of hypertension in the range 140-160/90-100 mm Hg. mandatory (SOMANZ 2014).

In decision of the XVI Russian Forum "Mother and Child" attention is drawn to the importance not only of absolute indicators of blood pressure in pregnant women, but also to a relative increase in blood pressure compared to the baseline, especially in women with hypotension (Decision of the XVI Russian Forum 2015, 131).

The benefits of antihypertensive treatment of pregnant women include not only reducing the risk of severe hypertension, but also preventing pregnancy complications such as uteroplacental blood flow disorders, fetal hypoxia, fetal growth retardation, placental abruption, premature birth of a low-birth-weight infant. Very high blood pressure or its significant variability are the cause of disorders of the uteroplacental circulation and placental abruption. In this case, antenatal fetal death, uteroplacental apoplexy (Couvelaire's uterus) and subsequent unavoidable hysterectomy may occur. Therefore, antihypertensive therapy prevents severe hypertension and at the same time prevents severe complications for the mother and fetus.

High blood pressure is the most noticeable and quickly observed symptom of pre-eclampsia. Sometimes in women with preeclampsia, blood pressure does not reach high values or blood pressure is variable, this causes management errors and an unfavorable outcome (Volkov et al. 2017, 5). In Russia, 176 cases of maternal mortality associated with preeclampsia were analyzed, only 41% of women had hypertension, and 44% of women had critical hypertension with a blood pressure of 170/110 mm Hg. and higher. In 6.3% of women with eclampsia, blood pressure was no higher than 140-145/100 mm Hg (Sidorova et al. 2013, 37). Later similar findings again confirmed (Sidorova et al. 2015, 13-14).

The level of hypertension for the start of drug therapy is the subject of discussion. In accordance with current guidelines of the European Society of Cardiology (ESC) and the European Society of Hypertension (ESH) for patients with chronic arterial hypertension, gestational hypertension or organ dysfunction, when blood pressure is> 140/90 mmHg. drug treatment should be prescribed (2018 ESC/ESH, 3080). Calcium channel blockers, methyldopa, labetalol are the drugs of choice according to the recommendations of ESC/ESH 2018.Intravenous urapidil, labetalol and nicardipine can be used for women with severe pre-eclampsia who have hypertension SBP ≥170 mmHg or DBP ≥110 mmHg. For women with severe pre-eclampsia complicated by pulmonary edema, nitroglycerin (glyceryl trinitrate) is the drug of choice.

Current recommendations do not contain data on the threshold level of blood pressure to start the use of antihypertensive drugs. Experts have a common opinion about the need for antihypertensive treatment in all women with blood pressure ≥160/110 mm Hg because there is a high risk of intracerebral hemorrhage and eclampsia. On the other hand, blood pressure is ≥ 160/110 mm Hg in combination with organ dysfunction meets the criterion of severe pre-eclampsia, which is an indication for childbirth. Labetalol, nifedipine is recommended for the first line of antihypertensive drugs, hydralazine, diazoxide are recommended for the second line. Prolonged use of atenolol and other highly selective β-blockers is associated with fetal growth retardation.

So, the use of calcium channel blockers and labetalol in the treatment of hypertension in pregnant women is common to the recommendations of all experts in the world.

Magnesium Sulphate

Magnesium sulphate was used for the first time in the early 20th century to treat eclampsia. Nowadays magnesium sulphate is recommended by WHO and is used worldwide.

The national clinical guideline of the United Kingdom recommended a full intravenous or intramuscular course of magnesium sulphate as the method of choice for both preventing eclampsia with severe pre-eclampsia and treating eclampsia based on information from the UK Obstetric Surveillance System (UKOSS) that a wide the spread of magnesium sulphate use explains the decrease in the frequency of eclampsia. Between February 2005 and February 2006, all women from 229 hospitals with maternity departments in the UK were included in the study. Results were obtained for 94% of women, eclampsia was in 2.7 cases per 10,000 births (Knight 2007, 1073), of which 99% received magnesium sulphate, 26% of patients had repeated convulsions, but no woman died (Knight 2007, 1075).

Cochrane systematic reviews for maternity showed great benefit of using magnesium sulphate for women with preeclampsia and eclampsia. Six trials with 11,444 women comparedmagnesiumsulphatewith placebo or no anticonvulsant and they demonstrated that magnesium sulphatereduces the risk of eclampsia (RR=0.41, 95% CI 0.29-0.58) (Duley, Gülmezoglu, Henderson-Smart et al. 2010, 26-27). Three trials with 397 women comparedmagnesiumsulphatewith lytic cocktail (chlorpromazine, promethazine and pethidine) in women with eclampsia. Magnesiumsulphatereduced maternal deaths (RR=0.14, 95% CI 0.03-0.59), prevent further seizures (RR 0.06, 95% CI 0.03-0.12) (Duley, Gülmezoglu and Chou 2010, 20). Seven trials compared magnesium sulphate and diazepam in women with eclampsia and confirmed the effect of magnesium sulphate for reduction of maternal death (RR=0.59, 95% CI 0.38-0.92 for 1396 women) and recurrence of seizures (RR 0.43, 95% CI 0.33-0.55 for 1390 women) (Duley, Henderson-Smart, Walker et al. 2010, 29).

The World Health Organization recommends magnesium sulfate for the prevention of eclampsia in women with severe pre-eclampsia, and prefers this medicine to other anticonvulsants based on high-quality evidence and a strong degree of persuasiveness (WHO 2011, 2). Progressive doctors urge specialists from all countries to use magnesium sulphate for the treatment of severe pre-eclampsia and eclampsia, as therapeutic and economic efficacy and safety have been proven for magnesium sulphate (Langer et al. 2008, 705).

Consensus

To make a decision on the general objective principles of pre-eclampsia management, the working group of the International Society for the Study of Hypertension in Pregnant Women has evaluated definitions, classifications, preventive measures and treatment recommendations in existing national and international guidelines on clinical practice (CPGs) for hypertensive disorders in pregnancy. The experts selected documents from various databases published for 10 years and only from English-speaking countries. Each document was evaluated by five experts. Six hundred ninety-five references were found and analyzed using the AGREE II method (Appraisal of Guidelines for Research and Evaluation) used by international experts to evaluate the methodological accuracy and clarity of practical guidelines.

Only 6 guidelines met AGREE II criteria: American College of Obstetrics and Gynecology,Society of Obstetricians and Gynaecologists of Canada, National Institute of Health and Care Excellence (UK), Queensland (Australia), Society of Obstetric Medicine of Australia and New Zealand, European Society of Cardiology (Bazzano A.N.et al, 2016). As a result, experts received a consensus on pre-eclampsia on the following items:

- Childbirth is a way out of pre-eclampsia. With pre-eclampsia, 37 weeks of gestation is optimal for childbirth, whereas with gestational hypertension, the pregnancy can be prolonged.
- Strict bed rest and injections of intravenous fluids should not be recommended for women with preeclampsia.
- In case of high blood pressure, antihypertensive drugs should be prescribed.
- In the antenatal period with premature pregnancy, corticosteroids should be prescribed to prevent respiratory distress syndrome of the newborn. It is also the prevention of other events related to the immaturity of the newborn, such as cerebral hemorrhages, necrotizing enterocolitis, mechanical ventilation and intensive care, neonatal death.
- It is necessary to prescribe magnesium sulfate for the treatment of eclampsia, as well as for the prevention of eclampsia in women with pre-eclampsia.

Unfortunately, there are no unified recommendations regarding the level of blood pressure for starting antihypertensive therapy, as well as for gestational age for prescribing corticosteroids for the purpose of antenatal prevention of respiratory distress syndrome.

CONSEQUENCES

Hypertensive disorders during pregnancy and pre-eclampsia significantly deteriorate the health of women in the future (Ying et al. 2018, 3). In the long-term prospective in women with a history of preeclampsia the risk of death is higher (OR 1.37, 95% CI 1.05-1.79) and associated with cardiovascular diseases (OR 2.53, 95% CI 1.28-4.99) (Ayansina et al. 2016, 347). The high risk of death in the long-term period for women with a history of hypertension during pregnancy was proven on a cohort of 31,656 women who gave birth at the Australian metropolitan hospital from January 1, 1980 to December 31, 1989. There were 4387 (14%) hypertensive women, of whom 129 in the following years died, while from normotensive 521 women died (OR 1.56; 95% CI 1.28-1.89; P < .001) (Tooher J. et al. 2016).

The risk of death from cardiovascular disease in the future in women with a history of pre-eclampsia depends on the parity of childbirth and the gestational age at which pre-eclampsia manifested.

The risk of cardiovascular death is higher in the long term after preterm preeclampsia (OR 9.4; 95% CI 6.5–13.7). This conclusion was obtained from two studies according to the Medical Birth Registry of Norway and the national Cause of Death Registry of a large group of women who gave birth in the period 1967-2002 (Skjaerven et al. 2012, e7677) and in the period 1980–2002 (HR, 2.8; 95% CI, 1.25–6.29) (Riise et al. 2017, e004158).

CONCLUSION

Pre-eclampsia is still a significant cause of maternal mortality in the world. Scientific studies have gained knowledge about the important role of angiogenic factors of preeclampsia. There are classic diagnostic criteria for preeclampsia. Currently, for the diagnosis of preeclampsia, international experts recommend to consider hypertension, signs of multiorgan dysfunction, and placental disorders. There are common recommendations for prescribing antihypertensive drugs for significant hypertension, corticosteroids for preterm pregnancy, magnesium sulfate for the prevention and treatment of eclampsia.

Childbirth is the only effective way to eliminate pre-eclampsia. However, with early preeclampsia and preterm delivery, there is a high risk of adverse outcome for the newborn.There is still no consensus on the level of hypertension for starting antihypertensive therapy and on gestational age for prescribing corticosteroids for the prevention of respiratory distress syndrome.

REFERENCES

[1] ACOG (American College of Obstetricians and Gynecologists),Society for Maternal-Fetal Medicine. 2017. *Obstetric Care consensus No. 6: Periviable Birth.* Obstetrics and gynecology130(4):e187-e199. https://doi.org/10.1097/AOG.0000000000002352.

[2] Ananth,Cande V.,Katherine M. Keyes, Ronald J. Wapner. 2013. "Pre-eclampsia rates in the United States, 1980-2010: age-period-cohort analysis." *British Medical Journal* 347:f6564. Published online 2013 Nov 7. https://doi.org/10.1136/bmj.f6564.

[3] Ayansina, D., C. Black, S.J. Hall, A.Marks, C.Millar, G.J.Prescott,K. Wilde, S. Bhattacharya. 2016. "Long term effects of gestational hypertension and pre-eclampsia on kidney function: Record linkage study." *Pregnancy Hypertension: An International Journal of Women's Cardiovascular Health* 6(4): 344-349. https://doi.org/10.1016/j.preghy.2016.08.231.

[4] Bazzano,Alessandra N,Erik Green,Anita Madison,Andrew Barton, Veronica Gillispie,Lydia A L Bazzano. 2016. "Assessment of the quality and content of national and international guidelines on hypertensive disorders of pregnancy using the AGREE II instrument." *BMJ Open* 6(1): e009189. Online issue publication January 18, 2016. https://doi.org/10.1136/bmjopen-2015-009189.

[5] Black, Carin, Fabricioda Silva Costa. 2018. "Biomarker Immunoassays in the Diagnosis of Preeclampsia: Calculating the sFlt1/PlGF Ratio Using the Cobas®e 411 Analyser." In *Preeclampsia. Methods in Molecular Biology,* edited by Padma Murthi, Cathy Vaillancourt, 9-26. New York: Humana Press. https://doi.org/10.1007/978-1-4939-7498-6_2.

[6] Churchill, David, Lelia Duley, Jim G. Thornton, Mahmoud Moussa, Hind SM Ali, Kate F. Walker. 2018. "Interventionist versus expectant care for severe pre-eclampsia between 24 and 34 weeks' gestation." *Cochrane Database of Systematic Reviews* 10. Art. No.: CD003106. https://doi.org/10.1002/14651858.CD003106.pub3.

[7] Coviello, Elizabeth M., Sara N. Iqbal, Katherine L. Grantz, Chun-Chih Huang, Helain J. Landy, Uma M. Reddy. 2019. "Early preterm preeclampsia outcomes by intended mode of delivery." *American Journal of Obstetrics and Gynecology* 220, no. 1(January): 100.e1-100.e9. https://doi.org/10.1016/j.ajog.2018.09.027.

[8] [Decision of the XVI Russian Forum "Mother and Child," Moscow, September 22-25, 2015.*Akusherstvoiginekologiya/Obstetrics and gynecology* 10: 130-132. (in Russian)].

[9] Duhig, Kate E., Jenny Myers, Paul T. Seed, Jenie Sparkes, Jessica Lowe, Rachael M. Hunter, Andrew H. Shennan, Lucy C. Chappell. 2019. "Placental growth factor testing to assess women with suspected pre-eclampsia: a multicentre, pragmatic, stepped-wedge cluster-randomised controlled trial." *Lancet*393:1807–18. http://dx.doi.org/10.1016/S0140-6736(18)33212-4.

[10] Duley, Lelia, A. MetinGülmezoglu, David J. Henderson-Smart, Doris Chou. 2010. "Magnesium sulphate and other anticonvulsants for women with pre-eclampsia." *Cochrane Database of Systematic Reviews.* 11, Art. No.: CD000025. https://doi.org/10.1002/14651858.CD000025.pub2.

[11] Duley, Lelia, A. MetinGülmezoglu, Doris Chou. 2010. "Magnesium sulphate versus lytic cocktail for eclampsia." *Cochrane Database of Systematic Reviews.* 9, Art. No.: CD002960. https://doi.org/10.1002/14651858.CD002960.pub2.

[12] Duley, Lelia, David J. Henderson-Smart, Godfrey J.A. Walker, Doris Chou. 2010. "Magnesium sulphate versus diazepam for eclampsia." *Cochrane Database of Systematic Reviews.* 12, Art. No.: CD000127. https://doi.org/10.1002/14651858.CD000127.pub2.

[13] Ehrenfest, Hugo. 1920. "Recent literature on eclampsia: A critical review."*American Journal of Obstetrics and Gynecology* 1(2): 214–218. https://doi.org/10.1016/S0002-9378(20)90191-6.

[14] Figueira, Sarah Franco, Cyril Wolf, Marisa D'Innocenzo, João Paulo VeneziandeCarvalho, Mariana Granado Barbosa, Eduardo Zlotnik, Eduardo Cordioli. 2018. "Economic evaluation of sFlt-1/PlGF ratio test in pre-eclampsia prediction and diagnosis in two Brazilian

hospitals." *Pregnancy Hypertension: An International Journal of Women's Cardiovascular Health* 13:30-36. https://doi.org/10.1016/j.preghy.2018.04.014.

[15] Knight M. on behalf of UKOSS. 2007. "Eclampsia in the United Kingdom 2005." *BJOG An International Journal of Obstetrics & Gynaecology*.114: 1072-8. https://doi.org/10.1111/j.1471-0528.2007.01423.x.

[16] Langenveld, Josje, Anita C. J. Ravelli, Anton H. van Kaam, David P. van der Ham, Maria G. van Pampus, Martina Porath, Ben Willem Mol, Wessel Ganzevoort. 2011. "Neonatal outcome of pregnancies complicated by hypertensive disorders between 34 and 37 weeks of gestation: a 7 year retrospective analysis of a national registry." *American Journal of Obstetrics and Gynecology* 205, no. 6(December): 540.e1-540.e7.https://doi.org/10.1016/j.ajog.2011.07.003.

[17] Langer, Ana, José Villar, Katie Tell, Theresa Kim, Stephen Kennedy. 2008. "Reducing eclampsia-related deaths—a call to action."*Lancet*371, no. 9614 (March):705–6. https://doi.org/10.1016/S0140-6736(08)60321-9.

[18] Lowe, Sandra A.,Lucy Bowyer, Karin Lust, Lawrence P. McMahon, Mark R. Morton, Robyn A. North, Michael J. Paech, Joanne M. Said. 2015. "The SOMANZ Guidelines for the Management of Hypertensive Disorders of Pregnancy 2014." *Australian and New Zealand Journal of Obstetrics and Gynaecology*55(1):11-6. https://doi.org/10.1111/ajo.12253.

[19] Magee, Laura A., Anouk Pels, Michael Helewa, Evelyne Rey, Peter von Dadelszen. 2014. "Diagnosis, evaluation, and management of the hypertensive disorders of pregnancy." *Pregnancy Hypertension: An International Journal of Women's Cardiovascular Health* 4, no. 2 (April): 105-45. http://dx.doi.org/10.1016/j.preghy.2014.01.003.

[20] Nathan, Hannah L., Paul T. Seed, Natasha L. Hezelgrave, Annemarie De Greeff, Elodie Lawley, John Anthony, David R. Hall, Wilhelm Steyn, Lucy C. Chappell, Andrew H. Shennan. 2018. "Early warning system hypertension thresholds to predict adverse outcomes in pre-

eclampsia: A prospective cohort study." *Pregnancy Hypertension: An International Journal of Women's Cardiovascular Health*12:183–188. https://doi.org/10.1016/j.preghy.2017.11.003.

[21] Riise, Hilde Kristin Refvik, Gerhard Sulo, Grethe S. Tell, Jannicke Igland, Ottar Nygard, Stein Emil Vollset, Ann-Charlotte Iversen, Rigmor Austgulen, Anne Kjersti Daltveit. 2017. "Incident Coronary Heart Disease After Preeclampsia: Role of Reduced Fetal Growth, Preterm Delivery, and Parity." *Journal of the American Heart Association*6, no. 3 (March): e004158. https://doi.org/10.1161/JAHA.116.004158.

[22] Rysavy, Matthew A., Lei Li, Edward F. Bell, Abhik Das, Susan R. Hintz, Barbara J. Stoll, Betty R. Vohr, Waldemar A. Carlo et al. 2015. "Between-hospital variation in treatment and outcomes in extremely preterm infants [published correction appears in *The New England journal of medicine*372, no. 25:2469].*The New England journal of medicine*372, no. 19(May):1801–1811. https://doi.org/10.1056/NEJMoa1410689.

[23] Say, Lale, Doris Chou, Alison Gemmill, Özge Tunçalp, Ann-Beth Moller, Jane Daniels, A Metin Gülmezoglu, Marleen Temmerman, Leontine Alkema. 2014. "Global causes of maternal death: a WHO systematic analysis." *The Lancet Global Health* 2, no. 6 (May): e323 - e333. http://dx.doi.org/10.1016/ S2214-109X(14)70227-X.

[24] Schneuer, Francisco J., Natasha Nassar, Cyrille Guilbert, Vitomir Tasevski, Anthony W. Ashton, Jonathan M. Morris, Christine L. Roberts. 2013. "First trimester screening of serum soluble fms-like tyrosine kinase-1 and placental growth factor predicting hypertensive disorders of pregnancy." *Pregnancy Hypertension: An International Journal of Women's Cardiovascular Health*3, no. 4 (October):215–221. http://dx.doi.org/10.1016/j.preghy.2013.04.119.

[25] Shennan,Andrew H., Marcus Green, Lucy C. Chappell. 2017. "Maternal deaths in the UK: pre-eclampsia deaths are avoidable." *The Lancet* 389, no.10069 (February):582-584. https://doi.org/10.1016/S0140-6736(17)30184-8.

[26] Sibai, Baha M.2011. "Evaluation and management of severe preeclampsia before 34 weeks' gestation." *American Journal of Obstetrics and Gynecology* 205(3): 191-198. https://doi.org/10.1016/ j.ajog.2011.07.017.

[27] [Sidorova I.S., Milovanov A.P., Nikitina N.A., Bardachova A.V., Rzaeva A.A. 2013. "Severe preeclampsia and eclampsia: critical conditions for the mother and fetus." *Akusherstvoiginekologiya/ Obstetrics and gynecology* 12: 34-40. (in Russian)].

[28] [Sidorova I.S., Filippov O.S., Nikitina N.A., Guseva E.V. 2015. "Causes of maternal mortality from preeclampsia and eclampsia in Russia in 2013." *Akusherstvoiginekologiya/Obstetrics and gynecology* 4: 11-17. (in Russian)].

[29] Skjaerven, Rolv, Allen J. Wilcox, Kari Klungsøyr, Lorentz M.Irgens, BjørnEgilVikse, Lars J.Vatten, RolvTerje Lie. 2012. "Cardiovascular mortality after pre-eclampsia in one child mothers: prospective, population based cohort study." *British Medical Journal* 345(November):e7677. https://doi.org/10.1136/bmj.e7677.

[30] SOMANZ (Society of Obstetric Medicine of Australia and New Zealand). 2014. "Guidelines for the Management of Hypertensive Disorders of Pregnancy." Accessed June 19. https://www.somanz. org/downloads/HTguidelineupdatedJune2015.pdf.

[31] Task Force on Hypertension in Pregnancy. Report of the American College of Obstetricians and Gynecologists'. 2013. "Hypertension in pregnancy: executive summary." *Obstetrics and gynecology* 122(5): 1122-31. https://doi.org/ 10.1097/01.AOG.0000437382.03963.88.

[32] Thornton, Charlene, Hannah Dahlen, Andrew Korda, Annemarie Hennessy. 2013. "The incidence of preeclampsia and eclampsia and associated maternal mortality in Australia from population-linked datasets: 2000-2008." *American Journal of Obstetrics and Gynecology* 208, no. 6(June): 476.e1-476.e5. https://doi.org/ 10.1016/j.ajog.2013.02.042.

[33] Tooher, Jane, Charlene Thornton, Angela Makris, Robert Ogle, Andrew Korda, John Horvathd,Annemarie Hennessy. 2016. "Hypertension in pregnancy and long-term cardiovascular mortality:

a retrospective cohort study." *American Journal of Obstetrics and Gynecology* 214 no. 6(June):722.e1-722.e6. https://doi.org/10.1016/j.ajog.2015.12.047.

[34] [Volkov V.G., Granatovich N.N., Survillo E.V., Cherepenko O.V. 2017. "Retrospective analysis of maternal mortality in preeclampsia and eclampsia." *Rossiyskiyvestnikakushera-ginekologa/The Russian bulletin of the obstetrician-gynecologist* 3: 4-8. https://doi.org/10.17116/rosakush20171734-8. (in Russian)].

[35] WHO Recommendations for Prevention and Treatment of Pre-Eclampsia and Eclampsia. 2011. *Geneva: World Health Organization.* ISBN-13:978-92-4-154833-5.Available from: https://www.ncbi.nlm.nih.gov/books/NBK140561/.

[36] Ying, Wendy, Janet M. Catov, Pamela Ouyang. 2018. "Hypertensive Disorders of Pregnancy and Future Maternal Cardiovascular Risk."*Journal of the American Heart Association*7, no. 17 (September):e009382. https://doi.org/10.1161/JAHA.118.009382.

[37] Younge, Noelle, Ricki F. Goldstein, Carla M. Bann, Susan R. Hintz, Ravi M. Patel, P. Brian Smith, Edward F. Bell et al. 2017. "Survival and Neurodevelopmental Outcomes among Periviable Infants." *The New England journal of medicine*376, no. 7 (February):617-28. https://doi.org/10.1056/NEJMoa1605566.

[38] 2018 ESC/ESH Guidelines for the management of arterial hypertension. The Task Force for the management of arterial hypertension of the European Society of Cardiology (ESC) and the European Society of Hypertension (ESH). 2018. *European Heart Journal* 39, no. 33 (September):3021-3104. https://doi.org/10.1093/eurheartj/ehy339.

BIOGRAPHICAL SKETCH

Alena I Baranouskaya

Affiliation: Belarusian State Medical University, Minsk, Belarus
Education: Vitebsk State Medical University, Vitebsk, Belarus

Business Address: Dzerzhinski Ave., 83, Minsk, Republic of Belarus, 220116

Research and Professional Experience: Obstetrics. Pathology of pregnant women. Perinatology

Professional Appointments: Doctor obstetrician-gynecologist. Doctor of Medical Sciences. Professor of the Department of Obstetrics and Gynecology

Publications from the Last 3 Years:

1) [Baranouskaya, Alena I., OlgaA. Lositskaya, A.S. Sofonova. 2016. "Specific features of the fetoplacental complex in hypertensive women." *Zdravoohranenie/Healthcare*2:26-30. (in Russian)].
2) [Znovets, Tatyana V., Siarhei V. Zhavaranak, Alena I. Baranouskaya, A.A. Arabey. 2016. "Hepatitis E in pregnant women with liver disease in the Republic of Belarus." *Zdravoohranenie/Healthcare*5:9-15. (in Russian)].
3) [Baranouskaya, Alena I., Marina A. Kustova, Siarhei V. Zhavaranak. 2016. "Features of HPV-infection in HIV-infected pregnant women." *Immunopatologiya, allergologiya, infektologiya/Immunopathology, allergology, infectology*1:50-56. https://doi.org/10.14427/jipai.2016.1.50 (in Russian)].
4) [Znovets, Tatyana V., Alena I. Baranouskaya, Siarhei V. Zhavaranak, E.A. Goshkevich, T.A. Zenovko. 2017. "Social and behavioral characteristics of modern HCV-infected women."

Reproduktivnoezdorov'e.VostochnayaEvropa/Reproductive Health.Eastern Europe 7, no. 5:779-781. (in Russian)].
5) [Baranouskaya, Alena I. 2017. "Hypertension in pregnancy and preeclampsia."*Meditsinskienovosti/Medical news*6:4-7. (in Russian)].
6) [Znovets, Tatyana V., Alena I. Baranouskaya, Siarhei V. Zhavaranak, L.A. Anisko, E.A. Goshkevich, I.L. Shiptenko. 2017. "Viral hepatitis C, first detected in pregnancy." *Immunopatologiya, allergologiya, infektologiya/Immunopathology, allergology, infectology*2:15-23. https://doi.org/10.14427/jipai.2017.2.15 (in Russian)].
7) [Znovets, Tatyana V., Siarhei V. Zhavaranak,Alena I. Baranouskaya, Y.O. Kuznetsov, Ivan A. Znovets, A.V. Ataman. 2018. "Clinical-biochemical characteristics and indirect liver fibrosis markers in HCV-infected pregnant women." *Immunopatologiya, allergologiya, infektologiya/Immunopathology, allergology, infectology*3:13-18. https://doi.org/10.14427/jipai.2018.3.13 (in Russian)].
8) [Znovets, Tatyana V., Alena I. Baranouskaya, Siarhei V. Zhavaranak, Ivan A. Znovets. 2018. "Perinatal outcome of HCV-infection." *Medicinskijzhurnal/ Medical journal*4:57-61. (in Russian)].
9) [Baranouskaya, Alena I. 2018. "Ectopia of gestational sac and heterotopic pregnancy." *Meditsinskienovosti/Medical news*4:9-11. (in Russian)].
10) [Baranouskaya, Alena I. 2018. "Preeclampsia in actual obstetrics." *Akusherstvoiginekologiya/Obstetrics and gynecology*11:5-9. (in Russian)].
11) [Baranouskaya, Alena I., Aleksandr V. Fedoseyenko, Aliaksandr.V. Krasnitski. 2018. "Heterotopic pregnancy in a natural conception cycle and delivery at term." *Rossiyskiyvestnikakushera-ginekologa/The Russian bulletin of the obstetrician-gynecologist* 18(6):70-72. (in Russian)].

BIBLIOGRAPHY

101 questions and answers about hypertension
LCCN	2011014362
Type of material	Book
Main title	101 questions and answers about hypertension / William M. Manger ... [et al.].
Edition	2nd ed.
Published/Created	Alameda, CA: Hunter House, 2011.
Description	xviii, 222 p.: ill.; 22 cm.
ISBN	9780897935715 (pbk.)
	0897935713 (pbk.)
LC classification	RC685.H8 M277 2011
Variant title	One hundred and one questions and answers about hypertension
	One hundred one questions and answers about hypertension
Related names	Manger, William Muir, 1920-
	Manger, William Muir, 1920- 100 questions and answers about hypertension.
Summary	"Hypertension, or high blood pressure, affects an estimated 50 million Americans and is a

major contributor to cardiovascular disease, the leading cause of death in the United States. Through proper management the effects of hypertension can be minimized. Dr. William Manger's 101 Questions & Answers About Hypertension is a comprehensive Q&A format book providing the reader all the information they need to help manage hypertension and prevent its often lethal effects. 101 Questions & Answers About Hypertension answers all the most important questions about hypertension and its relationship to other diseases, from hypothyroidism and Alzheimer's to arteriosclerosis and preeclampsia, among others. It also has suggestions for positive lifestyle changes as well as information on alternative and traditional treatment options and questions related to change of life and the effectiveness of blood pressure machines in pharmacies, shopping malls, etc. Question 8 addresses the enormous magnitude of hypertension in the United States. Hypertension is a precursor to stroke and cardiovascular disease. Cardiovascular disease kills nearly 1 million Americans every year and cripples and disables the same; it's also responsible for more than 52 million lost workdays. In addition, every year more than one-million people suffer heart attacks and 600,000 suffer strokes, a large percentage of both proving fatal. However, Dr. Manger is convinced these statistics can be reduced. Inspired by the decrease in the incidence of heart attack and stroke, Manger saw that with improved medical management and healthy lifestyle changes, hypertension could be controlled and its complications minimized or prevented. He believes a close patient-doctor relationship and a clear understanding of what hypertension is and how to manage it is essential for bringing it under control and minimizing the risk of further health complications. Even though Manger is positive overall about statistics, still there is room for improvement: nearly 30% of people suffering from hypertension go undiagnosed and only 27% of the 50 million people with this condition have their blood pressure under control. 101 Questions & Answers About Hypertension seeks to reduce the statistical gap by giving readers a comprehensive understanding of hypertension so they are able to knowledgeably communicate with their doctors and make informed decisions and choices to improve their health and reduce health risk"-- Provided by publisher.

"101 Questions & Answers About Hypertension is a comprehensive Q&A format book providing the reader all the information they need to help manage hypertension and prevent its often lethal effects. 101 Questions & Answers About Hypertension answers all the most important questions about hypertension and its relationship to other diseases, from hypothyroidism and Alzheimer's to arteriosclerosis and preeclampsia, among others. It also has suggestions for positive lifestyle changes as well as information on alternative and traditional treatment options and

	questions related to change of life and the effectiveness of blood pressure machines in pharmacies, shopping malls, etc"-- Provided by publisher.
Subjects	Hypertension--Miscellanea.
	Hypertension--Popular works.
Notes	Rev. ed. of: 100 questions and answers about hypertension / by William M. Manger and Ray W. Gifford, Jr. c2001.
	Includes bibliographical references and index.

Advances in fetal and neonatal physiology: proceedings of the Center for Perinatal Biology 40th Anniversary Symposium

LCCN	2014941729
Type of material	Book
Meeting name	Advances in Fetal and Neonatal Physiology (Symposium) (2013: Loma Linda, Calif.)
Main title	Advances in fetal and neonatal physiology: proceedings of the Center for Perinatal Biology 40th Anniversary Symposium / Lubo Zhang, Charles A. Ducsay, editors.
Published/Produced	New York: Springer, [2014]
	©2014
Description	xx, 245 pages: illustrations (some color), tables; 24 cm.
ISBN	9781493910304 (hbk.: alk. paper)
	1493910302 (hbk.: alk. paper)
LC classification	RG610 .A37 2014
Portion of title	Proceedings of the Center for Perinatal Biology 40th Anniversary Symposium
Related names	Zhang, Lubo, editor.
	Ducsay, Charles Andrew, 1953- editor.
	Loma Linda University. Center for Perinatal Biology, issuing body.

Summary

"To celebrate the Center for Perinatal Biology's 40th Anniversary, an illustrious group gathered at Loma Linda University in February 2013. That gathering of experts and this volume of the proceedings are a tribute to the founder of the Center, Lawrence D. Longo, M.D. These chapters present contributions from individuals who in some way or another were influenced by Dr. Longo. Covering a wide range of topics, and illustrating the diversity of thinking and scientific interests, these proceedings address basic science through to clinical problems in the developmental programming of health and disease"--Publisher's description.

Contents

"Surprised by joy": four decades of contributions to developmental physiology -- Lawrence D. Longo -- sGC-cGMP signaling: target for anticancer therapy -- Lawrence D. Longo: from chronic fetal hypoxia to proteomic predictors of fetal distress syndrome: a life devoted to research and mentoring based on virtue-ethics -- Pregnancy programming and preeclampsia: identifying a human endothelial model to study pregnancy-adapted endothelial function and endothelial adaptive failure in preeclamptic subjects -- Regulation of amniotic fluid volume: evolving concepts -- gestational diabetes, preeclampsia and cytokine release: similarities and differences in endothelial cell function -- Heart disease link to fetal hypoxia and oxidative stress -- Fetal breathing movements and changes at birth -- From fetal physiology to gene therapy: it all started in Loma Linda -- 30+ years of exercise in pregnancy -- Gap junction regulation of vascular tone: implications of modulatory intercellular communication during gestation -- Effect of preeclampsia on placental function: influence of sexual dimorphism, microRNA's and mitochondria -- Altitude, attitude and adaptation -- The separation of sexual activity and reproduction in human social evolution -- The influence of growth hormone on bone and adipose programming -- The fetal cerebral circulation: three decades of exploration by the LLU Center for Perinatal Biology -- Placental vascular defects in compromised pregnancies: effects of assisted reproductive technologies and other maternal stressors -- How to build a healthy heart from scratch -- Estrogen in the fetus -- Calcitonin gene related family peptides: importance in normal placental and fetal development.

Subjects   Loma Linda University. Center for Perinatal Biology.
Fetus--Physiology--Congresses.
Newborn infants--Physiology--Congresses.
Perinatology--Congresses.
Fetus--physiology--Congresses.
Infant, Newborn--physiology--Congresses.
Perinatology--Congresses.
Fetal Development--physiology--Congresses.
Pregnancy Complications--physiopathology--Congresses.
Fetus--Physiology.

Form/Genre   Conference proceedings.
Notes   This 40th Anniversary Symposium was held at the Center for Perinatal Biology of Loma Linda

	University, California on Feburary 11, 2013.
	Includes bibliographical references and index.
Additional formats	Print version: Advances in fetal and neonatal physiology. New York, NY: Springer, 2014 9781493910311 (OCoLC)884437972
Series	Advances in experimental medicine and biology, 0065-2598; 814
	Advances in experimental medicine and biology; v. 814. 0065-2598

Biomarkers of kidney disease

LCCN	2016948632
Type of material	Book
Uniform title	Biomarkers in kidney disease.
Main title	Biomarkers of kidney disease / edited by Charles L. Edelstein, MD, PhD, Division of Renal Diseases and Hypertension, University of Colorado Denver, Aurora, CO, United States.
Edition	Second edition.
Published/Produced	Amsterdam; Boston: Elsevier/Academic Press, [2017]
Description	xvii, 613 pages: illustrations; 24 cm
ISBN	9780128030141
	0128030143
LC classification	RC904 .B56 2017
Related names	Edelstein, Charles L. (Charles Louis), editor.
Contents	Chapter 1: Characteristics of an Ideal Biomarker of Kidney Diseases / M.R Bennett aand P. Devarajan -- Chapter 2: Statistical Considerations in Analysis and Interpretation of Biomarker Studies / C.R. Parikh and H. Theissen Philbrook -- Chapter 3: The Role of Metabolomics in the Study of Kidney Diseases and in the Development of Diagnostic Tools /

Bibliography

U. Christians, J. Klawitter, J. Klepacki and J. Klawitter -- Chapter 4: The Role of Proteomics in the Study of Kidney Diseases and in the Development of Diagnostic Tools / U. Christians, J. Klawitter, J. Klepacki and J. Klawitter -- Chapter 5: Cystatin C as a Multifaceted Biomarker in Kidney Disease and Its Role in Defining "Shrunken Pore Syndrome" / A. Grubb -- Chapter 6: Biomarkers in Acute Kidney Injury / C.L. Edelstein -- Chapter 7: Biomarkers of Extra-Renal Complications of AKI / S. Faubel -- Chapter 8: Biomarkers in Kidney Transplantation / S. Jain and A. Jani -- Chapter 9: Biomarkers of Renal Cancer / N.S. Vasudev and R.E. Banks -- Chapter 10: Proteomics and Advancements in Urinary Biomarkers of Diabetics Kidney Disease / M.L. Merchant and J.B. Klein -- Chapter 11: Biomarkers of Cardiovascular Risk in Chronic Kidney Disease / Z.H. Endre and R.J. Walker -- Chapter 12: Diagnostic and Prognostic Biomarkers in Autosomal Dominant Polycystic Kidney Disease / G. Fick-Brosnahan and B.Y. Reed -- Chapter 13: Biomarkers in Glomerular Disease / J.M. Arthur, E. Elnagar and N. Karakala -- Chapter 14: Biomarkers in Preeclampsia / S.A. Karamanchi.

Subjects Kidneys--Diseases--Molecular diagnosis.
Biochemical markers.
Kidney Diseases--diagnosis.
Biomarkers.

Notes Preceded by Biomarkers in kidney disease / edited by Charles L. Edelstein. 2011.
Includes bibliographical references and index.

Chesley's hypertensive disorders in pregnancy

LCCN	2009001376
Type of material	Book
Main title	Chesley's hypertensive disorders in pregnancy / edited by Marshall D. Lindheimer, James M. Roberts, F. Gary Cunningham.
Edition	3rd ed.
Published/Created	Amsterdam; Boston: Academic Press/Elsevier, c2009.
Description	x, 422 p., [8] p. of plates: ill. (some col.); 29 cm.
Links	Table of contents http://bvbr.bib-bvb.de:8991/F?func=service&doc_library=BVB01&doc_number=017738636&line_number=0001&func_code=DB_RECORDS&service_type=MEDIA
ISBN	9780123742131 (alk. paper) 0123742137 (alk. paper)
LC classification	RG580.H9 C48 2009
Portion of title	Hypertensive disorders in pregnancy
Related names	Lindheimer, Marshall D., 1932- Roberts, James M., 1941- Cunningham, F. Gary. Chesley, Leon C., 1908-2000.
Contents	Introduction, history, controversies, and definitions / Marshall D. Lindheimer ... [et al.] -- The clinical spectrum of preeclampsia / F. Gary Cunningham, James M. Roberts and Marshall D. Lindheimer -- Epidemiology of pregnancy-related hypertension / Roberta B. Ness and James M. Roberts -- Genetic factors in the etiology of preeclampsia/eclampsia / Kenneth Ward and Marshall D. Lindheimer -- The placenta in normal pregnancy and

preeclampsia / Susan J. Fisher, Michael McMaster and James M. Roberts -- Angiogenesis and preeclampsia / S. Ananth Karumanchi, Isaac E. Stillman and Marshall D. Lindheimer -- Metabolic syndrome and preeclampsia / Carl A. Hubel and James M. Roberts -- Immunology of normal pregnancy and preeclampsia / Christopher W.G. Redman, Ian L. Sargent, and James M. Roberts -- Endothelial cell dysfunction and oxidative stress / Robert N. Taylor, Sandra T. Davidge and James M. Roberts -- Animal models / Rocco C. Venuto and Marshall D. Lindheimer -- Tests to predict preeclampsia / Agustin Conde-Agudelo, Roberto Romero and Marshall D. Lindheimer. --Prevention of preeclampsia and eclampsia / Baha M. Sibai and F. Gary Cunningham -- Cerebrovascular (patho)physiology in preeclampsia/eclampsia / Gerda G. Zeeman, Marilyn J. Cipolla and F. Gary Cunningham -- Cardiovascular alterations in normal and preeclamptic pregnancy / Judith U. Hibbard, Sanjeev G. Shroff and Marshall D. Lindheimer -- Normal and abnormal volume homeostasis / Friedrich C. Luft, Eileen D.M. Gallery and Marshall D. Lindheimer -- Agonistic autoantibody-mediated disease / Ralf Dechend, Friedrich C. Luft and Marshall D. Lindheimer -- The kidney in normal pregnancy and preeclampsia / Kirk P. Conrad, Lillian W. Gaber and Marshall D. Lindheimer -- Platelets, coagulation, and the liver / Louise Kenny, Philip N. Baker and F. Gary Cunningham -- Chronic hypertension and pregnancy / Phyllis

	August and Marshall D. Lindheimer -- Antihypertensive treatment / Jason G. Umans, Edgardo J. Abalos and Marshall D. Lindheimer -- Management / Kenneth J. Leveno and F. Gary Cunningham.
Subjects	Hypertension in pregnancy. Eclampsia--physiopathology. Pre-Eclampsia--physiopathology. Hypertension--complications. Pregnancy Complications, Cardiovascular--physiopathology. Pregnancy.
Notes	Includes bibliographical references and index.

Chesley's Hypertensive disorders in pregnancy

LCCN	2015458416
Type of material	Book
Main title	Chesley's Hypertensive disorders in pregnancy / edited by Robert N. Taylor, MD, PHD; James M. Roberts, MD; F. Gary Cunningham, MD; Marshall D. Lindheimer, MD.
Edition	Fourth Edition.
Published/Produced	Amsterdam; Boston: Elsevier/AP, Academic Press is an imprint of Elsevier, [2015]
Description	x, 473 pages: illustrations (some color); 29 cm
Links	Publisher description http://www.loc.gov/catdir/enhancements/fy1606/2015458416-d.html
ISBN	9780124078666 0124078664
LC classification	RG580.H9 C48 2015
Portion of title	Hypertensive disorders in pregnancy
Related names	Taylor, Robert N., 1953- editor. Roberts, James M., 1941- editor. Cunningham, F. Gary, editor.

Contents

Lindheimer, Marshall D., 1932-, editor.
Chesley, Leon C., 1908-2000.
Introduction, history, controversies, and definitions / Marshall D. Lindheimer, Robert N. Taylor, James M. Roberts, F. Gary Cunningham, and Leon Chelsey -- The clinical spectrum of preeclampsia / F. Gary Cunningham, James M. Roberts, and Robert N. Taylor -- Epidemiology of pregnancy-related hypertension / Janet W. Rich-Edwards, Roberta B. Ness, and James M. Roberts -- Genetic factors in the etiology of preeclampsia/eclampsia / Kenneth Ward and Robert N. Taylor -- The placenta in normal pregnancy and preeclampsia / Susan J. Fisher, Michael McMaster and James M. Roberts -- Angiogenesis and preeclampsia / S. Ananth Karumanchi, Sarosh Rana, and Robert N. Taylor -- Metabolic syndrome and preeclampsia / Arun Jeyabalan, Carl A. Hubel, and James M. Roberts -- Immunology of normal pregnancy and preeclampsia / Christopher W.G. Redman, Ian L. Sargent, and Robert N. Taylor -- Endothelial cell dysfunction / Sandra T. Davidge, Christianne J.M. de Groot, and Robert N. Taylor -- Animal models for investigating pathophysiological mechanisms of preeclampsia / Joey P. Granger, Eric M. George, and James M. Roberts -- Tests to predict preeclampsia / Agustin Conde-Agudelo, Roberto Romero, and James M. Roberts -- Prevention of preeclampsia and eclampsia / Anne Cathrine Staff, Baha M. Sibai, and F. Gary Cunningham -- Cerebrovascular pathophysiology in

preeclampsia and eclampsia / Marilyn J. Cipolla, Gerda G. Zeeman, and F. Gary Cunningham -- Cardiovascular alterations in normal and preeclamptic pregnancy / Judith U. Hibbard, Sanjeev G. Shroff, and F. Gary Cunningham -- The renin-angiotensin system, its autoantibodies, and body fluid volume in preeclampsia / Ralf Dechend, Babette LaMarca, and Robert N. Taylor -- The kidney and normal pregnancy and preeclampsia / Kirk P. Conrad, Isaac E. Stillman, and Marshall D. Lindheimer -- Platelets, coagulation, and the liver / Louise C. Kenny, Keith R. McCrae, and F. Gary Cunningham -- Chronic hypertension and pregnancy / Phyllis August, Arun Jeyabalan, and James M. Roberts -- Antihypertensive treatment / Jason G. Umans, Edgardo J. Abalos, and F. Gary Cunninghma -- Clinical management / James M. Alexander and F. Gary Cunningham.

Subjects — Hypertension in pregnancy.
Notes — Includes bibliographical references and index.

Chronic kidney disease and hypertension
LCCN — 2014955206
Type of material — Book
Main title — Chronic kidney disease and hypertension / Matthew R. Weir, Edgar V. Lerma, editors.
Published/Produced — New York: Humana Press, [2015]
Description — xiii, 257 pages: illustrations (some color); 24 cm
ISBN — 9781493919819 (alk. paper)
1493919814 (alk. paper)
LC classification — RC918.R4 C468 2015

Related names   Weir, Matthew R., 1952- editor.
Lerma, Edgar V., editor.

Summary   The treatment of hypertension has become the most important intervention in the management of all forms of chronic kidney disease. Chronic Kidney Disease and Hypertension is a current, concise, and practical guide to the identification, treatment and management of hypertension in patients with chronic kidney disease. In depth chapters discuss many relevant clinical questions and the future of treatment through medications and or novel new devices. Written by expert authors, Chronic Kidney Disease and Hypertension provides an up-to-date perspective on management and treatment and how it may re-shape practice approaches tomorrow. -- Source other than Library of Congress.

Contents   Changes in Guideline Trends and Applications in Practice: JNC 2013 and the future -- Central BP monitoring, Home BP Monitoring, Ambulatory BP Monitoring in CKD -- Resistant hypertension in patients with chronic kidney disease -- Neurogenic Factors In Hypertension Associated With Chronic Kidney Disease -- Novel Molecules -- Dual Inhibitors: RAAS Blockers/Combination Therapies: What Do All These Trials Mean? -- Renal Sympathetic Denervation -- Novel baroreceptor activation therapy -- Blood Pressure Vaccines -- Masked Hypertension: Does it Lead to CVD or CKD? -- White Coat Hypertension- Do We Really Understand It Now? -- Uric Acid And Hypertension -- Is There Really A Link?.-

	Preeclampsia: Angiogenic factors, blood pressure, and the kidney -- Inflammation and Hypertension -- Genome-Wide Association Studies (Gwas) Of Blood Pressure In Different Populations -- Endocrine Hypertension and Chronic Kidney Disease -- Hypertension in Children with Chronic Kidney Disease -- Obesity/OSA/Metabolic syndrome in pts with CKD and hypertension-the missing link.
Subjects	Chronic renal failure.
	Medicine.
	Cardiology.
	Nephrology.
	Renal Insufficiency, Chronic--etiology.
	Hypertension, Renal--complications.
	Cardiology.
	Medicine.
	Nephrology.
Notes	Includes bibliographical references and index.
Series	Clinical hypertension and vascular diseases
	Clinical hypertension and vascular diseases.

Clinical anesthesiology: lessons learned from morbidity and mortality conferences

LCCN	2013954905
Type of material	Book
Main title	Clinical anesthesiology: lessons learned from morbidity and mortality conferences / Jonathan L. Benumof, editor.
Published/Produced	New York: Springer, [2014]
Description	xxxii, 563 pages: illustrations; 24 cm.
ISBN	9781461486954 (pbk.: alk. paper)
	1461486955 (pbk.: alk. paper)
	(eBook)

Bibliography

LC classification	RD81 .C5835 2014
Related names	Benumof, Jonathan, 1942- editor.
Summary	The book presents more than 60 real-life cases which together memorably and succinctly convey the depth and breadth of clinical anesthesiology. Each chapter includes a case summary, questions, lessons learned, and selected references. Tables and distinctive visual synopses of key teaching points enhance many chapters. The cases have been selected by Dr. Benumof from the Morbidity and Mortality (M & M) conferences of the Department of Anesthesiology, University of California, San Diego, which he has moderated the last several years, and residents and junior faculty have crafted them into the chapters of this book. Structured in a novel way, the UCSD Anesthesiology M&Ms maximize teaching and learning, and these cases bring that experience right to the reader's finger tips. Case coverage of respiration- and circulation-related problems, obstetrics, neurology, pain and regional anesthesia, pediatrics, outpatient surgery, and special topics Resource for anesthesiology and critical care medicine trainees Review tool for board certification or recertification Fun reading - valuable lessons!-- Source other than Library of Congress.
Contents	Respiration-related cases -- Cannot ventilate, cannot intubate due to airway hemorrhage -- Pulmonary edema following attempted nasal intubation for mandibular fracture repair -- Loss of critical airway -- Anterior mediastinal mass -- Awake intubation with a NIM tube: how is it

done? -- Hemodynamic collapse following a mainstem intubation -- Hypoxemia during tracheostomy -- Anesthetic depth and mask ventilation in the prone position -- Jet ventilation through a cookgas airway exchange catheter -- End of case evaluation and management of a patient post airway mass excision -- Possible recurrent laryngeal nerve injury -- Obstructive sleep apnea, and dead in bed -- Bilevel positive air pressure, decreased sensorium, aspiration and capnography -- Perioperative management of a patient previously treated with bleomycin undergoing thoracic surgery -- Intra-operative airway fire -- Obesity hypoventilation syndrome -- Circulation-related cases -- Hemorrhage during endovascular repair of thoracic aorta -- Pacemakers and automatic implantable cardioverter defibrillators -- Acute myocardial infarction during laparoscopic surgery -- Sickle cell and preeclampsia -- Dysrhythmias in a patient with Crohn's disease -- Hematologic disorders: hemophilia and disseminated intravascular coagulation -- Blood transfusion and the Jehovah's Witness patient -- Cardiac and pulmonary contusions -- Intraoperative coagulopathy -- Hypotension in chronic methamphetamine user -- Venous air embolism during arteriovenous malformation repair -- Cardiac tamponade -- Case of intraoperative new-onset atrial fibrillation -- Valvular disease -- Obstetrics-related cases -- Labor epidural with unrecognized dural puncture, causing high sensory block, hypotension, fetal bradycardia and post dural puncture headache -- Acute pulmonary dysfunction immediately after cesarean delivery under general anesthesia -- Jehovah's Witness with placenta previa and increta for cesarean hysterectomy -- A pregnant patient with mitral stenosis -- Unrecognized uterine hyperstimulation due to oxytocin and combined spinal-epidural analgesia -- Super morbidly obese patient for elective repeat cesarean section -- Probable amniotic fluid embolus -- Emergent cesarean section -- Pregnancy plus atrial septal defect vs Eisenmenger Syndrome -- Uterine abruption -- Pediatric-related cases -- Neonatal resuscitation following spontaneous vaginal delivery -- Anxious, coughing and bound to obstruct -- Special diseases/conditions/situations -- Hypothermia during laparoscopic nephrectomy -- Operating room management case scenarios -- Anaphylaxis reactions -- Autonomic dysreflexia -- Porphyrias -- Monitored anesthesia care: medical implications; and wrong-sided operations: legal implications -- Diabetic ketoacidosis in the urgent anesthesia setting -- Fever, altered mental status, and rigidity in the perioperative course -- Neuro/neuromuscular-related cases -- Emergent craniotomy for evacuation of epidural hematoma -- Hyperkalemia and residual neuromuscular blockade after kidney transplantation -- A defasciculating dose of nondepolarizing neuromuscular blocker -- Postoperative monocular vision loss -- Delayed emergence after aneurysm clipping -- Pain and

	regional anesthesia related cases -- Unintentional dural puncture in a patient with severe preeclampsia -- Complex regional pain syndrome -- Vascular absorption of local anesthetic producing systemic toxicity -- Inadvertent high spinal in parturient -- Outpatient surgery-related cases -- Plastic surgery in a surgeon's office -- Orthopedic surgery in an ambulatory surgicenter -- Eye surgery at an outpatient surgicenter -- Endoscopic sinus surgery at an outpatient sugicenter.
Subjects	Medicine.
	Anesthesiology.
	Anesthesia--adverse effects.
	Intraoperative Complications--prevention & control.
	Patient Harm--prevention & control.
	Anesthesiology.
	Medicine.
Form/Genre	Case Reports.
Notes	Includes bibliographical references and indexes.
Additional formats	Online version: Clinical anesthesiology. New York: Springer, ©2014 9781461486961 (OCoLC)867819952

Diabetes in women

LCCN	2009926313
Type of material	Book
Main title	Diabetes in women / edited by Agathocles Tsatsoulis, Jennifer Wyckoff, Florence M. Brown.
Published/Created	Totowa, N.J.: Humana; London: Springer [distributor], c2009.

Description	xii, 461 p.: ill. (chiefly col.); 27 cm.
Links	Inhaltsverzeichnis http://bvbr.bib-bvb.de:8991/F?func=service&doc_library=BVB01&doc_number=018950288&line_number=0001&func_code=DB_RECORDS&service_type=MEDIA
ISBN	9781603272490 (cased: alk. paper)
	1603272496 (cased: alk. paper)
	160327250X (ebk.)
	9781603272506 (ebk.)
LC classification	RC660 .D4495 2009
Related names	Tsatsoulis, Agathocles.
	Wyckoff, Jennifer Ann.
	Brown, Florence M., 1957-
Contents	Sex differences in energy balance, body composition, and body fat distribution / André Tchernof -- Menopause and diabetes mellitus / Emily D. Szmuilowicz and Ellen W. Seely -- Cardiovascular disease in women with diabetes / Sonia Gajula, Ashwini Reddy, L. Romayne ...[et al] -- Insulin resistance, diabetes, and cardiovascular risk in women and the paradigm of the polycystic ovary syndrome / Renato Pasquali and Alessandra Gambineri -- Developmental programming of polycystic ovary syndrome: role of prenatal androgen excess / Agathocles Tsatsoulis -- An anthropological view of the impact of poverty and globalization on the emerging epidemic of obesity / Patricia Aguirre -- Eating disorders and depression in women with diabetes / Patricia A. Colton and Gary Rodin -- Sexual health in women with diabetes / Andrea Salonia, Roberto Lanzi, Emanuele Bosi ...[et al] -- Contraception for women with diabetes / Siri

L. Kjos -- The effect of PCOS on fertility and pregnancy / Kelsey E.S. Salley and John E. Nestler -- The effect of pregnancy on energy metabolism, body composition, and endothelial function / Dilys J. Freeman and Naveed Sattar -- The epidemiology of diabetes in women and the looming epidemic of GDM in the third world / S.M. Sadikot -- Gestational diabetes mellitus: diagnosis, maternal and fetal outcomes, and management / Assiamira Ferrara and Catherine Kim -- Nutrition and pregnancy / Jo-Anne M. Rizzotto, Judy Giusti, and Laurie Higgins -- Preconception care for women with diabetes mellitus / Howard Blank and Jennifer Wyckoff -- Obstetric care of the woman with diabetes / Tamara C. Takoudes -- Medical management of preexisting diabetes in pregnancy / Angelina L. Trujillo, Lorena Wright, and Lois Jovanovic -- Use of ultrasound in the metabolic management of gestational diabetes and preexisting diabetes mellitus in pregnancy / Schaefer-Graf UM -- Preeclampsia / Allison L. Cohen and S. Ananth Karumanchi -- The infant of the diabetic mother: metabolic imprinting / Janet K. Snell-Bergeon and Dana Dabelea -- The genetic basis of diabetes / Hui-Qi Qu and Constantin Polychronakos -- Breastfeeding and diabetes / Julie Scott Taylor, Melissa Nothnagle, and Susanna R. Magee -- Management of disease in women with diabetes / Catherine Kim.

Subjects   Diabetes in women.
Diabetes Mellitus--physiopathology.
Diabetes Mellitus--therapy.
Women's Health.

Notes	Includes bibliographical references and index.
Series	Contemporary diabetes
	Contemporary diabetes.

Evidence-based obstetrics and gynecology

LCCN	2018041057
Type of material	Book
Uniform title	Evidence-based obstetrics and gynecology (Norwitz)
Main title	Evidence-based obstetrics and gynecology / edited by Errol R. Norwitz, Carolyn M. Zelop, David A. Miller, David Keefe.
Published/Produced	Hoboken, NJ: Wiley, 2018.
ISBN	9781444334333 (hardback)
LC classification	RG101
Related names	Norwitz, Errol R., editor.
	Zelop, Carolyn M., editor.
	Miller, David A. (David Arthur), 1961- editor.
	Keefe, David (David L.), editor.
Summary	"The most comprehensive evidence-based guide to both obstetrics and gynecology Aimed at practicing obstetricians, gynecologists, and trainees in the specialty, Evidence-based Obstetrics and Gynecology concentrates on the clinical practice areas of diagnosis, investigation and management. The first section of the book discusses evidence-based medicine methodology in the context of the two specialties. The second and third sections cover all the major conditions in obstetrics and gynecology, with each chapter reviewing the best available evidence for management of the particular condition. The chapters are structured in line with EBM methodology, meaning the

cases generate the relevant clinical questions.Evidence-based Obstetrics and Gynecology provides in-depth chapter coverage of abnormal vaginal bleeding; ectopic pregnancy; pelvic pain; lower genital tract infections; contraception and sterilization; breast diseases; urogynecology; endocrinology and infertility; puberty and precocious puberty; cervical dysplasia and HPV; cervical, vaginal, vulvar, uterine, and ovarian cancer; preconception care; prenatal care and diagnosis; drugs and medications in pregnancy; maternal complications; chronic hypertension; diabetes mellitus; thyroid disease; neurologic disease; psychiatric disease; postterm pregnancy; fetal complications; preeclampsia; and more. First book to address evidence-based practice for obstetrics and gynecology combinedEBM is a highly relevant approach for this high risk specialtyEdited by leading US specialist involved in the evidence-based medicine movementEvidence-Based Obstetrics and Gynecology is an important text for obstetricians and gynecologists in practice and in training, as well as for specialist nurses"--Provided by publisher.

Subjects	Genital Diseases, Female
	Pregnancy Complications
	Evidence-Based Medicine
Notes	Includes bibliographical references and index.
Additional formats	Online version: Hoboken, NJ: Wiley, 2018 9781119072928 (DLC) 2018041689

Evidence-based obstetrics and gynecology
LCCN 2018041689
Type of material Book
Uniform title Evidence-based obstetrics and gynecology (Norwitz)
Main title Evidence-based obstetrics and gynecology / edited by Errol R. Norwitz, Carolyn M. Zelop, David A. Miller, David Keefe.
Published/Produced Hoboken, NJ: Wiley, 2018.
Description 1 online resource.
ISBN 9781119072928 (Adobe PDF)
9781119072959 (ePub)
LC classification RG101
Related names Norwitz, Errol R., editor.
Zelop, Carolyn M., editor.
Miller, David A. (David Arthur), 1961- editor.
Keefe, David (David L.), editor.
Summary "The most comprehensive evidence-based guide to both obstetrics and gynecology Aimed at practicing obstetricians, gynecologists, and trainees in the specialty, Evidence-based Obstetrics and Gynecology concentrates on the clinical practice areas of diagnosis, investigation and management. The first section of the book discusses evidence-based medicine methodology in the context of the two specialties. The second and third sections cover all the major conditions in obstetrics and gynecology, with each chapter reviewing the best available evidence for management of the particular condition. The chapters are structured in line with EBM methodology, meaning the cases generate the relevant clinical questions.Evidence-based Obstetrics and

	Gynecology provides in-depth chapter coverage of abnormal vaginal bleeding; ectopic pregnancy; pelvic pain; lower genital tract infections; contraception and sterilization; breast diseases; urogynecology; endocrinology and infertility; puberty and precocious puberty; cervical dysplasia and HPV; cervical, vaginal, vulvar, uterine, and ovarian cancer; preconception care; prenatal care and diagnosis; drugs and medications in pregnancy; maternal complications; chronic hypertension; diabetes mellitus; thyroid disease; neurologic disease; psychiatric disease; postterm pregnancy; fetal complications; preeclampsia; and more. First book to address evidence-based practice for obstetrics and gynecology combinedEBM is a highly relevant approach for this high risk specialtyEdited by leading US specialist involved in the evidence-based medicine movementEvidence-Based Obstetrics and Gynecology is an important text for obstetricians and gynecologists in practice and in training, as well as for specialist nurses"-- Provided by publisher.
Subjects	Genital Diseases, Female
	Pregnancy Complications
	Evidence-Based Medicine
Notes	Includes bibliographical references and index.
Additional formats	Print version: Hoboken, NJ: Wiley, 2018 9781444334333 (DLC) 2018041057

Evolutionary medicine and health: new perspectives

LCCN	2007016223
Type of material	Book

Main title	Evolutionary medicine and health: new perspectives / [edited by] Wenda R. Trevathan, E.O. Smith, James J. McKenna.
Published/Created	New York: Oxford University Press, 2008.
Description	xii, 532 p.: ill.; 25 cm.
Links	Table of contents only http://www.loc.gov/catdir/toc/ecip0716/2007016223.html
ISBN	9780195307061 (pbk.: alk. paper) 9780195307054 (hardcover: alk. paper)
LC classification	RB152 .E963 2008
Related names	Trevathan, Wenda. Smith, Euclid O. McKenna, James J. (James Joseph), 1948-
Contents	An overview of evolutionary medicine / Wenda Trevathan, E. O. Smith, and James J. McKenna -- Human evolution, diet, and nutrition: when the body meets the buffet / Bethany L. Turner ... [et al.] -- Diabesity and Darwinian medicine: the evolution of an epidemic / Leslie Sue Lieberman -- To eat, or what not to eat: a critique of the official Norwegian dietary guidelines / Iver Mysterud ... [et al.] -- Cow's milk consumption and health: an evolutionary perspective / Andrea S. Wiley -- Not by bread alone: the role of psychosocial stress in age at first reproduction and in health inequalities / James S. Chisholm and David A. Coall -- Early life effects on reproductive function / Alejandra Núñez-de la Mora and Gillian R. Bentley -- Impaired reproductive function in women in western and westernizing populations: an evolutionary approach / Tessa M. Pollard and Nigel Unwin -- Should women menstruate? an evolutionary perspective on menstrual-

suppressing oral contraceptives / Lynnette Leidy Sievert -- An evolutionary perspective on premenstrual syndrome: implications for investigating infectious causes of chronic disease / Caroline Doyle, Holly A. Swain Ewald, and Paul W. Ewald -- The possible role of eclampsia/preeclampsia in the evolution of human reproduction / Pierre-Yves Robillard ... [et al.] -- Breastfeeding and mother-infant sleep proximity: implications for infant care / Helen Ball and Kristin Klingaman -- Why words can hurt us: social relationships, stress, and health / Mark V. Flinn -- Why are we vulnerable to acute mountain sickness? / Cynthia M. Beall -- Evolution and modern behavioral problems: the case of addiction / Daniel H. Lende -- After dark: the evolutionary ecology of human sleep / Carol M. Worthman -- Evolutionary medicine and obesity: developmental adaptive responses in human body composition / Jack Baker ... [et al.] -- The developmental origins of adult health: intergenerational inertia in adaptation and disease / Christopher W. Kuzawa -- An evolutionary perspective on the causes of chronic diseases: atherosclerosis as an illustration / Paul W. Ewald -- Genes, geographic ancestry, and disease susceptibility: applications of evolutionary medicine to clinical settings / Douglas E. Crews and Linda M. Gerber -- From ancient seas to modern disease: evolution and congestive heart failure / E. Jennifer Weil -- Evolution at the intersection of biology and medicine / Stephen Lewis -- The importance of evolution for medicine /

	Randolph M. Nesse.
Subjects	Diseases--Causes and theories of causation.
	Human evolution.
	Medicine--Philosophy.
	Disease--etiology--Essays.
	Evolution--Essays.
	Epidemiologic Factors--Essays.
	Humans--Essays.
	Philosophy, Medical--Essays.
Notes	Includes bibliographical references (p. 441-522) and index.

Fertility and pregnancy: an epidemiologic perspective
LCCN	2009025396
Type of material	Book
Personal name	Wilcox, Allen J.
Main title	Fertility and pregnancy: an epidemiologic perspective / Allen J. Wilcox.
Published/Created	Oxford; New York: Oxford University Press, 2010.
Description	xii, 324 p.: ill., maps; 25 cm.
ISBN	9780195342864 (alk. paper)
	0195342860 (alk. paper)
LC classification	QP252 .W55 2010
Review	"Fertility and Pregnancy: An Epidemiologic Perspective offers an overview of human reproduction - how it works, and what causes it to go wrong. Weaving together history, biology, obstetrics, pediatrics, demography, infectious diseases, molecular genetics, and evolutionary biology, Allen Wilcox brings a fresh coherence to the epidemiologic study of reproduction and pregnancy. Along the way, he provides entertaining anecdotes, superb graphs, odd

Contents	tidbits, and occasional humor that bring the topic to life."--BOOK JACKET. The creative biology of human reproduction -- On getting pregnant -- How humans control their fertility -- Infections and reproduction -- The genetics of reproduction -- Evolutionary biology and eugenics -- Heterogeneity of risk -- Reproductive epidemiology: themes and variations -- Fertility and fecundability -- Early pregnancy loss -- Miscarriage -- Stillbirth and infant mortality -- Twins and more -- Gestational age and preterm delivery -- Birth weight and fetal growth -- Birth defects -- Sex ratio -- Maternal mortality and morbidity -- Preeclampsia -- Fetal exposures and adult disease -- Unanswered questions in reproductive epidemiology.
Subjects	Human reproduction. Reproductive health. Infertility--Epidemiology. Pregnancy--Complications--Epidemiology. Fertility. Pregnancy Complications--epidemiology. Reproductive Physiological Phenomena.
Notes	Includes bibliographical references and index.

Genetic diagnoses

LCCN	2011018627
Type of material	Book
Main title	Genetic diagnoses / editor, Radha Jonnalagedda Sarma.
Published/Created	Hauppauge, N.Y.: Nova Science Publishers, c2011.
Description	xi, 202 p.: ill.; 26 cm.

ISBN	9781613248669 (hardcover)
LC classification	RB155.6 .G4613 2011
Related names	Sarma, Radha Jonnalagedda.
Contents	Defining a cause: result priority between preeclampsia and thyroid function / Ioannis Katsakoulas, Clio P. Mavragani -- Molecular diagnosis of thalassemia / Wen Wang, Boran Jiang, Samuel S. Chong -- Fuzzy logic and the least squares method in diagnosis problem solving / Alexander P. Rotshtein, Hanna B. Rakytyanska -- Molecular diagnosis of spinocerebellar ataxias / Laia Rodriguez-Revenga ... [et al.] -- Genetics of left ventricular noncompaction / Radha J. Sarma -- A genetic diagnosis to type 1 diabetes / Jose Luis Santiago, Laura Espino-Paisan, Elena Urcelay -- State of the heart on genetics of congenital heart diseases: molecular basis, genetic diagnosis, and counselling / Giuseppe Limongelli ... [et al.].
Subjects	Human chromosome abnormalities--Diagnosis. Molecular biology. Genetic Testing. Genetic Counseling. Genetic Techniques. Molecular Biology.
Notes	Includes bibliographical references and index.

Handbook of clinical laboratory testing during pregnancy

LCCN	2003023726
Type of material	Book
Main title	Handbook of clinical laboratory testing during pregnancy / edited by Ann M. Gronowski; foreword by Gillian Lockitch.
Published/Created	Totowa, N.J.: Humana Press, c2004.

Description	xvii, 454 p.: ill.; 26 cm. + 1 CD-ROM (4 3/4 in.)
Links	Table of contents http://www.loc.gov/catdir/toc/ecip0410/2003023726.html Book review (E-STREAMS) http://www.e-streams.com/es0802/es0802_3927.html Publisher description http://www.loc.gov/catdir/enhancements/fy0825/2003023726-d.html
ISBN	1588292703 (alk. paper) 1592597874 (E-ISBN)
LC classification	RG527.5.L3 H36 2004
Related names	Gronowski, Ann M.
Contents	Human pregnancy: an overview / Ann M. Gronowski -- Human chorionic gonadtropin / Laurence A. Cole -- Biological markers of preterm delivery / Stephen F. Thung and Alan M. Peaceman -- Markers of fetal lung maturity / Edward R. Ashwood -- Maternal prenatal screening for fetal defects / Andrew R. MacRae and Jacob A. Canick -- Chromosome analysis in prenatal diagnosis / Syed M. Jalal, Adewale Adeyinka, and Alan Thornhill -- Diagnosis and monitoring of ectopic and abnormal pregnancies / Gary Lipscomb -- Thyroid disease during pregnancy: assessment of the mother / Corinne R. Fantz and Ann M. Gronowski -- Thyroid disease during pregnancy: assessment of the fetus / Pratima K. Singh and Ann M. Gronowski -- Hematology and hemostasis during pregnancy / Charles Eby -- Hemolytic disease of the newborn / David G. Grenache -- Prenatal screening and diagnosis of congenital infection / Lynn Bry -- Laboratory testing for group B streptococcus in the pregnant patient / Sebastian

	Faro -- Immunologic diseases of pregnancy / William A. Bennett -- Recurrent pregnancy loss / Carolyn B. Coulam -- Multifetal gestations / Isaac Blickstein and Louis G. Keith -- Diabetes in pregnancy / Jonathan W. Dukes, Albert C. Chen, and Lois Jovanovic -- Preeclampsia, eclampsia, and hypertension / Kee-Hak Lim and Melanie M. Watkins -- Liver diseases in pregnancy / Jason D. Wright and Yoel Sadovsky.
Subjects	Obstetrics--Diagnosis--Handbooks, manuals, etc.
Prenatal diagnosis--Handbooks, manuals, etc.
Fetus--Diseases--Diagnosis--Handbooks, manuals, etc.
Pregnancy--Complications--Diagnosis--Handbooks, manuals, etc.
Diagnosis, Laboratory--Handbooks, manuals, etc.
Prenatal Diagnosis--methods--Handbooks.
Fetal Diseases--diagnosis--Handbooks.
Laboratory Techniques and Procedures--Handbooks.
Pregnancy Complications--diagnosis--Handbooks.
Notes	Includes bibliographical references and index.
Computer file info	System requirements for accompanying disk: Adobe Reader 6.0 or later.
Series	Current clinical pathology

Handbook of obstetric and gynecologic emergencies
LCCN	2005006351
Type of material	Book
Main title	Handbook of obstetric and gynecologic

	emergencies / edited by Guy I. Benrubi; with 42 contributors.
Edition	3rd ed.
Published/Created	Philadelphia: Lippincott Williams & Wilkins, c2005.
Description	xviii, 461 p.: ill.; 21 cm.
Links	Table of contents http://www.loc.gov/catdir/toc/ecip059/2005006351.html
	Publisher description http://www.loc.gov/catdir/enhancements/fy0712/2005006351-d.html
ISBN	0781762367 (alk. paper)
LC classification	RG571 .O245 2005
Related names	Benrubi, Guy I.
Contents	Medical emergencies in the pregnant patient / Saju Joy, Laura Hughes -- Acute abdominal pain in pregnancy / Richard Boothby -- Ectopic pregnancy / David Boyd, Andrew Kaunitz, & Catherine McIntyre -- Trauma in pregnancy / David Caro, Lynnette Doan-Wiggins -- Cardiopulmonary resuscitation during pregnancy / David Caro, Lynnette Doan-Wiggins -- Perimortem cesarean section / Deborah S. Lyon -- Hypertensive disorders of pregnancy: preeclampsia, eclampsia / Luis Sanchez-Ramos -- Bleeding in pregnancy / David C. Jones -- Infections in pregnancy / David C. Adair / Shawn P. Stallings -- Pregnancy women & chemical-biological warfare / Shawn P. Stallings, Joseph H. Kipikasa, and C. David Adair -- Mosquito borne illnesses: Western Nile virus / Zachary K. Thomas, C. David Adair, and Shawn P. Stallings -- Delivery in the emergency department / Isaac Delke -- Human

immunodeficiency virus infection and pregnancy: labor and delivery management / Isaac Delke -- Postpartum emergencies / David C. Jones -- Role of imaging modalities in obstetric emergencies / Francisco L. Gaudier and Tamara M. Metcalfe -- Drug therapy in pregnancy / Thanh T. Hogan ... [et al.] -- Complications of legal and illegal abortion / James L. Jones, Andrew M. Kaunitz -- Sexually transmitted diseases / I. Keith Stone -- Vulvar and vaginal diseases / Benson J. Horowitz -- Menorrhagia & abnormal vaginal bleeding / Deborah S. Lyon -- Pelvic mass / Boniface U. Ndubisi, Mitzi Brock and Jonathan Tammela -- Torsion of ovary / Charles J Dunton -- Oncologic emergencies / Guy I. Benrubi, Robert C. Nuss and Ann L. Harwood-Nuss -- Postoperative emergencies / Michael Callahan and Gregory Sutton -- Emergency evaluation and treatment of the sexual assault victim / James L. Jones and J.M. Whitworth -- Gynecologic traumas / Tracey Maurer -- Imaging in gynecologic emergencies / Marcia E. Murakami, Joseph Cernigliaro, and Maribel U. Lockwood -- Urogynecologic emergencies / Cheryl Iglesia and Alan Gehrich -- Emergency room communication issues: dealing with crisis / Marghani M. Reever and Deborah S. Lyon.

Subjects   Obstetrical emergencies--Handbooks, manuals, etc.
Gynecologic emergencies--Handbooks, manuals, etc.
Obstetrics.
Emergencies.

	Genital Diseases, Female.
	Pregnancy Complications.
Notes	Includes bibliographical references and index.

Heart disease in women

LCCN	2008041207
Type of material	Book
Main title	Heart disease in women / Benjamin V. Lardner and Harrison R. Pennelton, editors.
Published/Created	New York: Nova Science, c2009.
Description	xiii, 268 p.: ill.; 27 cm.
Links	Table of contents only http://www.loc.gov/catdir/toc/fy1001/2008041207.html
ISBN	9781606920664 (hardcover)
	1606920669 (hardcover)
LC classification	RC682 .H3836 2009
Related names	Lardner, Benjamin V.
	Pennelton, Harrison R.
Contents	Cardiac rehabilitation: secondary prevention of cardiovascular disease in women / Richard Snow ... [et al.] -- Effects of estrogen and its receptors on myocardial infraction / Jiang Hong ... [et al.] -- Preeclampsia and risk of cardiovascular disease: epidemiology and pathophysiology / Giovanna Oggè, Simona Cardaropoli, Tullia Todros -- Diabetes and the risk of coronary heart disease among women / Gang Hu -- The impact of heart rate as a cardiovascular risk / Taku Inoue, Kunitoshi Iseki -- Women in a world of men's disease: the case of female cardiac patients / Michal Rassin -- Thromboembolism and coronary heart disease: in which aspects are women different? / Sigrid Nikol, Katharina Middendorf -- Aging women

	and coronary heart disease / Marek A. Kosmicki, Hanna Szwed -- Prognosis of women with acute coronary syndromes: an overview / Andreja Sinkovic -- The effects of aging on the electrophysiological properties of the atrial myocardium in women with and without paroxysmal atrial fibrillation / Osmar Antonio Centurión, Akihiko Shimizu, Shojiro Isomoto -- Women and angina pectoris: emergency department and diagnostic difficulties in an undeveloped community / Esed Omerkic, Fahir Barakovic.
Subjects	Heart diseases in women.
	Heart Diseases.
	Women's Health.
Notes	Includes bibliographical references and index.

Hypertension in pregnancy

LCCN	2013022521
Type of material	Book
Corporate name	American College of Obstetricians and Gynecologists. Task Force on Hypertension in Pregnancy, author.
Main title	Hypertension in pregnancy / developed by the Task Force on Hypertension in Pregnancy.
Published/Produced	Washington, DC: American College of Obstetricians and Gynecologists, [2013] ©2013
Description	x, 89 pages; 28 cm
ISBN	9781934984284 (pbk.)
	1934984280 (pbk.)
LC classification	RG575.5 .A44 2013
Related names	American College of Obstetricians and Gynecologists, issuing body.

Contents	Classification of hypertensive disorders -- Establishing the diagnosis of preeclampsia and eclampsia -- Prediction of preeclampsia -- Prevention of preeclampsia -- Management of preeclampsia and HELLP syndrome -- Management of women with prior preeclampsia -- Chronic hypertension in pregnancy and superimposed preeclampsia -- Later-life cardiovascular disease in women with prior preeclampsia -- Patient education -- State of the science and research recommendations.
Subjects	Hypertension, Pregnancy-Induced--Practice Guideline.
Notes	Includes bibliographical references.

Hypertensive disease in pregnancy

LCCN	2014395234
Type of material	Book
Main title	Hypertensive disease in pregnancy / editors, Sabaratnam Arulkumaran, MD, PhD, DSc, FRCS, FRCOG, Professor Emeritus of Obstetrics and Gynecology, St George's University of London, Cranmer Terrance, London, United Kingdom, Sanjay A Gupte, Consultant Obstetrician and Gynecologist, Director, Gupte Hospital and Center for Research in Reproduction, Pune, Maharashtra, India, Evita Fernandez, Consultant Obstetrician and Managing Director, Fernandez Hospital Pvt Ltd, Hyderabad, Andhra Pradesh, India.
Edition	First edition.
Published/Produced	New Delhi; Philadelphia: Jaypee Brothers Medical Publishers (P) Ltd, 2014.
Description	xix, 171 pages: illustrations (some color); 26 cm

ISBN	9789350909515
	9350909510
LC classification	RG580.H9 H955 2014
Related names	Arulkumaran, Sabaratnam, editor.
	Gupte, Sanjay A., editor.
	Fernandez, Evita, editor.
Subjects	Hypertension in pregnancy.
	Preeclampsia.
	Hypertension, Pregnancy-Induced.
Notes	Includes bibliographical references and index.

Molecular approaches to reproductive and newborn medicine: a subject collection from Cold Spring Harbor perspectives in medicine

LCCN	2015009577
Type of material	Book
Main title	Molecular approaches to reproductive and newborn medicine: a subject collection from Cold Spring Harbor perspectives in medicine / edited by Diana W. Bianchi, Tufts University School of Medicine, Errol R. Norwitz, Tufts University School of Medicine.
Published/Produced	Cold Spring Harbor, New York: Cold Spring Harbor Laboratory Press, [2015]
Description	vii, 406 pages: color illustrations; 27 cm.
ISBN	9781621820895 (hardcover: alk. paper)
LC classification	RC889 .M72 2015
Related names	Bianchi, Diana W., editor.
	Norwitz, Errol R., editor.
Contents	MicroRNA in ovarian biology and disease / Lynda K. McGinnis, Lacey J. Luense, and Lane K. Christenson -- Confrontation, consolidation, and recognition: the oocyte's perspective on the incoming sperm / David Miller --

Intergenerational transfer of epigenetic information in sperm / Oliver J. Rando -- HOX genes and female reproduction / Hongling Du and Hugh S. Taylor -- Human endometrial transcriptomics: implications for embryonic implantation / E. Gomez, M. Ruiz-Alonso, Jose Miravet, and C. Simøn -- A molecular perspective on procedures and outcomes associated with assisted reproductive technologies / Monica A. Mainigi, Carmen Sapienza, Samantha Butts, and Christos Coutifaris -- Molecular cross-talk at the feto-maternal interface / Gendie E. Lash -- Placental extracellular vesicles and feto-maternal communication / M. Tong and L.W. Chamley -- The function of trophomirs and other microRNAs in the human placenta / Yoel Sadovsky, Jean-Francois Mouillet, Yingshi Ouyang, Avraham Bayer, and Carolyn B. Coyne -- The human placental methylome / Wendy P. Robinson and E. Magda Price -- The perinatal microbiome and pregnancy: moving beyond the vaginal microbiome / Amanda L. Prince, Derrick M. Chu, Maxim D. Seferovic, Kathleen M. Antony, Jun Ma, and Kjersti M. Aagaard -- Molecular regulation of parturition: a myometrial perspective / Nora E. Renthal, Koriand'r C. Williams, Alina P. Montalbano, Chien-Cheng Chen, Lu Gao, and Carole R. Mendelson -- Molecular regulation of parturition: the role of the "decidual clock" / Errol R. Norwitz, Elizabeth A. Bonney, Victoria V. Snegovskikh, Michelle A. Williams, Mark Phillippe, Joong Shin Park, and Vikki M.

Abrahams -- Genetic considerations in recurrent pregnancy loss / Kassie J. Hyde and Danny J. Schust -- Genomics of preterm birth / Kayleigh A. Swaggart, Mihaela Pavlicev, and Louis J. Muglia -- Molecular mechanisms of preeclampsia / Tammy Hod, Ana Sofia Cerdeira, and S. Ananth Karumanchi -- Effects of maternal obesity on fetal programming: molecular approaches / Caterina Neri, and Andrea G. Edlow -- Noninvasive prenatal screening for genetic diseases using massively parallel sequencing of maternal plasma DNA / Lyn S. Chitty and Y.M. Dennis Lo -- Noninvasive antenatal determination of fetal blood group using next generation sequencing / Klaus Rieneck, Frederik Banch Clausen, and Morten Hanefeld Dziegiel -- Genome-wide sequencing for prenatal detection of fetal single-gene disorders / Ignatia B. Van den Veyver and Christine M. Eng -- The amniotic fluid transcriptome as a guide to understanding fetal disease / Lillian M. Zwemer and Diana W. Bianchi -- Potential uses and inherent challenges of using genome-scale sequencing to augment current newborn screening / Jonathan Berg and Cynthia M. Powell -- Whole exome and whole genome sequencing in critically ill neonates suspected to have single gene disorders / Laurie D. Smith, Laurel K. Willig, and Stephen F. Kingsmore -- The neonatal salivary transcriptome / Jill L. Maron.

Subjects Reproductive Health--Collected Works.
Molecular Diagnostic Techniques--Collected Works.

	Neonatal Screening--Collected Works.
	Prenatal Diagnosis--Collected Works.
	Reproductive Techniques--Collected Works.
Notes	Includes bibliographical references and index.

Molecular mechanisms of preeclampsia

LCCN	96039273
Type of material	Book
Personal name	Arbogast, Bradley W., 1947-
Main title	Molecular mechanisms of preeclampsia / Bradley W. Arbogast, Robert N. Taylor.
Published/Created	New York: Chapman & Hall; Austin: R.G. Landes Co., c1996.
Description	203 p.: ill.; 26 cm.
ISBN	1570593973 (alk. paper)
	0412114712
LC classification	RG575.5 .A73 1996
Related names	Taylor, Robert N., 1953-
Subjects	Preeclampsia--Pathophysiology.
	Preeclampsia--Molecular aspects.
	Pre-Eclampsia.
Notes	Includes bibliographical references and index.
Series	Medical intelligence unit
	Medical intelligence unit (Unnumbered)

Obstetric anesthesia

LCCN	2010050965
Type of material	Book
Personal name	Palmer, Craig M., author.
Main title	Obstetric anesthesia / Craig M. Palmer, Robert D'Angelo, Michael J. Paech.
Published/Created	Oxford; New York: Oxford University Press, [2011], ©2011.
Description	xii, 427 pages: illustrations; 18 cm

ISBN	9780199733804 (pbk.: acid-free paper)
LC classification	RG732 .P36 2011
Related names	D'Angelo, Robert, author.
	Paech, Michael J., author.
Contents	Neuroanatomy and neurophysiology -- Anatomic and physiologic changes of pregnancy -- Pain relief for labor and delivery -- Anesthesia for cesarean delivery -- Post-cesarean analgesia -- Anesthesia for surgery during and after pregnancy -- Pregnancy induced hypertension and preeclampsia -- Obstetric hemorrhage -- Obesity -- Coexisting disease and other issues -- Complications of labor and delivery -- Fetal assessment and care -- Management of later complications of obstetric anesthesia and analgesia -- Critical care of the obstetric patient -- Neonatal resuscitation.
Subjects	Anesthesia in obstetrics.
	Analgesia.
	Anesthesia, Obstetrical.
	Analgesia, Obstetrical.
	Gynecologic Surgical Procedures--methods.
Notes	Includes bibliographical references and index.

Obstetric ultrasound: artistry in practice

LCCN	2007008365
Type of material	Book
Personal name	Hobbins, John C., 1936-
Main title	Obstetric ultrasound: artistry in practice / John C. Hobbins.
Published/Created	Malden, Mass: Blackwell Pub., 2008.
Description	ix, 195 p.: ill. (some col.); 26 cm.
Links	Table of contents only http://www.loc.gov/cat

Bibliography 121

	dir/toc/ecip0712/2007008365.html
	Contributor biographical information http://www.loc.gov/catdir/enhancements/fy0802/2007008365-b.html
	Publisher description http://www.loc.gov/catdir/enhancements/fy0802/2007008365-d.html
ISBN	9781405158152
LC classification	RG527.5.U48 H59 2008
Contents	Early pregnancy loss -- The placenta and umbilical cord -- Assessment of amniotic fluid -- Fetal biometry -- Intrauterine growth restriction -- Examination of the fetal cranium -- Examination of the fetal heart -- Fetal spine -- Fetal abdomen -- Fetal kidneys -- Fetal limbs -- Multiple gestations -- Advanced maternal age -- Diabetes -- Preeclampsia -- Preterm labor -- Rh disease (erythroblastosis fetalis) -- 3D and 4D ultrasound -- The safety of ultrasound -- The biophysical profile (BPP) -- Ultrasound on the labor and delivery floor -- The Hobbins take on various hot topics.
Subjects	Ultrasonics in obstetrics.
	Ultrasonography, Prenatal--methods.
	Embryonic Development.
	Fetal Development.
	Fetal Diseases--ultrasonography.
	Pregnancy--physiology.
	Pregnancy Complications--ultrasonography.
Notes	Includes bibliographical references and index.

Preeclampsia: basic, genomic, and clinical
LCCN	2018933025
Type of material	Book
Main title	Preeclampsia: basic, genomic, and clinical /

	[edited by] Shigeru Saito.
Published/Produced	New York, NY: Springer Berlin Heidelberg, 2018.
ISBN	9789811058905 (hard cover: alk. paper)

Pre-eclampsia: etiology and clinical practice

LCCN	2007002767
Type of material	Book
Main title	Pre-eclampsia: etiology and clinical practice / [edited by] Fiona Lyall, Michael Belfort.
Published/Created	Cambridge; New York: Cambridge University Press, 2007.
Description	xvii, 548 p.: ill.; 26 cm.
Links	Table of contents only http://www.loc.gov/cat dir/toc/ecip079/2007002767.html
	Publisher description http://www.loc.gov/catdir/ enhancements/fy0713/2007002767-d.html
	Contributor biographical information http:// www.loc.gov/catdir/enhancements/fy0803/2007 002767-b.html
ISBN	9780521831895 (hardback)
	052183189X (hardback)
LC classification	RG575.5 .P74 2007
Related names	Lyall, F.
	Belfort, Michael A., 1958-
Subjects	Preeclampsia.
	Pre-Eclampsia--etiology.
	Pre-Eclampsia--therapy.
Notes	Includes bibliographical references and index.

Pre-eclampsia: the facts: the hidden threat to pregnancy

LCCN	91031879
Type of material	Book
Personal name	Redman, Chris.

Main title	Pre-eclampsia: the facts: the hidden threat to pregnancy / Chris Redman and Isabel Walker.
Published/Created	Oxford; New York: Oxford University Press, 1992.
Description	x, 197 p.: ill.; 23 cm.
Links	Publisher description http://www.loc.gov/catdir/enhancements/fy0640/91031879-d.html
	Table of contents only http://www.loc.gov/catdir/enhancements/fy0640/91031879-t.html
ISBN	0192620126 (blb):
	0192620134 (plb):
LC classification	RG575.5 .R44 1992
Related names	Walker, Isabel.
Subjects	Preeclampsia.
	Pre-Eclampsia--popular works.
Notes	Includes index.
Series	Oxford medical publications

Preeclampsia and Eclampsia among Punjabi women: a haematological study

LCCN	2019328579
Type of material	Book
Main title	Preeclampsia and Eclampsia among Punjabi women: a haematological study / Zia Jamal.
Published/Produced	Delhi: Bookwell, 2019.
Description	xx, 215 pages

Pregnancy for dummies

LCCN	2008941625
Type of material	Book
Personal name	Stone, Joanne.
Main title	Pregnancy for dummies / by Joanne Stone, Keith Eddleman, and Mary Duenwald.
Edition	3rd ed.

Published/Created Hoboken, N.J.: Wiley Pub., c2009.
Description xx, 388 p.: ill.; 24 cm.
ISBN 047038767X (pbk.)
9780470387672 (pbk.)
LC classification RG525 .S735 2009
Related names Eddleman, Keith.
Duenwald, Mary.

Summary Offers all of the latest information expecting parents want to know, including expanded coverage on the health and well-being of both mother and child throughout pregnancy. Features new and updated coverage of prenatal genetic screening and diagnosis, amniocentesis, new high-tech ultrasounds, and the revised FDA/USDA food pyramid. It also discusses the recent celebrity trend of "on-demand" cesarean sections, multiple births, what to expect in labor and delivery, postpartum care, choosing bottle or breastfeeding, preparing a home (and siblings) for a new baby, caring for preemies, and the mother's mental as well as physical health.

Contents Introduction -- About this book -- What's new in this edition -- Conventions used in this book -- What you're not to read -- Foolish assumptions -- How this book is organized -- Part I. The game plan -- Part II. Pregnancy: a drama in three acts -- Part III. The big event: labor, delivery, and recovery -- Part IV. Dealing with special issues -- Part V. The part of tens -- Icons used in this book -- Where to go from here -- pt. 1. The game plan -- 1. From here to maternity -- Getting ready to get pregnant: the preconceptional visit -- Taking a look at your

Bibliography

history --Evaluating your current health -- Answering commonly asked questions -- Getting to your ideal body weight -- Reviewing your medications -- Considering nutritional supplements -- Recognizing the importance of vaccinations and immunity -- Quitting birth control -- Introducing sperm to egg: timing is everything -- Pinpointing ovulation -- Taking an effective (and fun) approach -- 2. I think I'm pregnant! -- Recognizing the signs of pregnancy -- Determining whether you're pregnant -- Getting an answer at home -- Going to your practitioner for answers -- Selecting the right practitioner for you -- Considering your options -- Asking questions before you choose -- Calculating your due date -- 3. Preparing for life during pregnancy -- Planning prenatal visits -- Preparing for physical and emotional changes -- Coping with mood swings -- Living through leg cramps -- Noticing vaginal discharge -- Putting up with backaches -- Handling stress -- Understanding the effects of medications, alcohol, and drugs on your baby -- Taking medications -- Smoking -- Drinking alcohol -- Using recreational/illicit drugs -- Looking at lifestyle changes -- Pampering yourself with beauty treatments -- Relaxing in hot tubs, whirlpools, saunas, or steam rooms -- Traveling -- Getting dental care -- Having sex -- Working during pregnancy: a different type of labor -- Considering occupational hazards -- Understanding pregnancy and the law -- 4. Diet and exercise for the expectant mother -- Looking at healthy weight gain -- Determining how much is enough -- Avoiding weight obsession -- Understanding your baby's weight gain -- Taking stock of what you're taking in -- Using the USDA Food Guide Pyramid -- Supplementing your diet -- Determining which foods are safe -- Eyeing potentially harmful foods -- Debunking popular food myths -- Considering special dietary needs -- Eating right, vegetarian-style -- Combating constipation -- Dealing with diabetes -- Working out for two -- Adapting to your body's changes -- Exercising without overdoing it -- Comparing forms of exercise. pt. II. Pregnancy: a drama in three acts -- 5. The first trimester -- A new life takes shape -- Adapting to how your body changes -- Breast changes -- Fatigue -- Any-time-of-day sickness -- Bloating -- Frequent urination -- Headaches -- Constipation -- Cramps -- Going to your first prenatal appointment -- Understanding the consultation -- Considering the physical exam -- Eyeing the standard tests -- Recognizing causes for concern -- Bleeding -- Miscarriage -- Ectopic pregnancy -- For dads: reacting to the news -- 6. The second trimester -- Discovering how your baby is developing -- Understanding your changing body -- Forgetfulness and clumsiness -- Gas -- Hair and nail growth -- Heartburn -- Lower abdominal/groin pain -- Nasal congestion -- Nose bleeds and bleeding gums -- Skin changes -- Checking in: prenatal visits -- Recognizing causes for concern -- Bleeding -- Fetal abnormality -- Incompetent cervix -- Knowing when to seek help -- For dads: watching mom grow -- 7. The third trimester -- Your baby gets ready for birth -- Movin' and shakin': fetal movements -- Flexing the breathing muscles -- Hiccupping in utero -- Keeping up with your changing body -- Accidents and falls -- Braxton-Hicks contractions -- Carpal tunnel syndrome -- Fatigue -- Hemorrhoids -- Insomnia -- Feeling the baby "drop" -- Pregnancy rashes and itches -- Preparing for breastfeeding -- Sciatica -- Shortness of breath -- Stretch marks -- Swelling -- Urinary stress incontinence -- Varicose veins -- Preparing for labor -- Making a birth plan -- Going back to school: classes to take -- Asking for a C-Section on demand -- Determining who's coming to the hospital -- Timing labor -- Using perineal massage -- Hitting the home stretch: prenatal visits in the third trimester -- Recognizing causes for concern -- Bleeding -- Breech presentation -- Decreased amniotic fluid volume -- Decreased fetal movement -- Fetal growth problems -- Leaking amniotic fluid -- Preeclampsia -- Preterm labor -- When the baby is late -- Getting ready to head to the hospital -- Packing your suitcase -- Choosing--and using--a car seat -- For dads--getting down to the wire -- 8. Understanding prenatal testing -- Considering tests for prenatal diagnosis in the first trimester -- Chorionic villus sampling -- Early amniocentesis -- Testing in the second trimester -- Second-trimester blood tests -- "Looking" at sound waves: ultrasound -- Testing with amniocentesis -- Other prenatal tests and procedures -- Looking at third-trimester tests --

Taking Group B strep cultures -- Gauging lung maturity -- Assessing your baby's current health -- 9. Checking your pregnancy week-by-week -- Weeks 0-4 -- Weeks 5-8 -- Weeks 9-12 -- Weeks 13-16 -- Weeks 17-20 -- Weeks 21-24 -- Weeks 25-28 -- Weeks 29-32 -- Weeks 33-36 -- Weeks 37-40 -- Weeks 40-42. pt. III. The big event: labor, delivery, and recovery -- 10. Honey, I think I'm in labor! -- Knowing When labor is real--and when it isn't -- Noticing changes before labor begins -- Discerning false labor from true labor -- Deciding when to call your practitioner -- Checking for labor with an internal exam -- Getting admitted to the hospital -- Settling into your hospital room -- Checking out the accommodations -- Monitoring your baby -- Fetal heart monitoring -- Other tests of fetal health -- Nudging things along: labor induction -- Elective induction -- Medically indicated induction -- Inducing labor -- Augmenting labor -- Getting the big picture: stages and characteristics of labor -- The first stage -- The second stage -- The third stage -- Handling labor pain -- Systemic medications -- Regional anesthetics -- General anesthesia -- Considering alternative birthing methods -- Delivering without anesthesia -- Giving birth at home -- Immersing yourself in a water birth -- 11. Special delivery: bringing your baby into the world -- Having a vaginal delivery -- Pushing the baby out -- Getting an episiotomy -- Handling prolonged second-stage labor -- The big moment: delivering your baby -- Delivering the placenta -- Repairing your perineum --

Bibliography

Assisting nature: operative vaginal delivery -- Having a cesarean delivery -- Understanding anesthesia -- Looking at reasons for cesarean delivery -- Recovering from a cesarean delivery -- Congratulations! You did it! -- Shaking after delivery -- Understanding postpartum bleeding -- Hearing your baby's first cry -- Checking your baby's condition -- Cutting the cord -- 12. Hello, world! Your newborn -- Looking at your bundle of joy -- Varnished in vernix -- The shape of the head -- Black-and-blue marks -- Blotches, patches, and more -- Baby hair -- Extremities -- Eyes and ears -- Genitalia and breasts -- Umbilical cord -- Newborn size -- Seeing how your baby breathes -- Knowing what to expect in the hospital -- Preparing baby for life outside the womb -- Understanding baby's developing digestive system -- Considering circumcision -- Spending time in the neonatal intensive care unit -- Checking in: baby's first doctor visit -- Considering heart rate and circulatory changes -- Looking at weight changes -- For dads: home at last--with the new family -- 13. Taking care of yourself after delivery -- Recuperating from delivery -- Looking and feeling like a new mom -- Understanding postpartum bleeding -- Dealing with perineal pain -- Surviving swelling -- Coping with your bladder -- Battling the hemorrhoid blues -- Understanding postpartum bowel function -- Continuing to recover at home -- Recovering from a cesarean delivery -- Going to the recovery room -- Taking it one step at a time -- Understanding post-cesarean pain -- Dealing with post-op pain -- Getting ready to go home -- Continuing to recover at home -- Going through more postpartum changes -- Sweating like a ... new mom -- Dealing with breast engorgement -- Understanding hair loss -- Chasing away the baby blues -- Recognizing postpartum depression -- Checking your progress: The first postpartum doctor visit -- Returning to "normal" life -- Getting fit all over again -- Losing the weight -- Pondering your postpartum diet -- Taking your vitamins -- Doing Kegel exercises -- Having sex again -- Choosing contraception -- 14. Feeding your baby -- Deciding between breast and bottle -- Sizing up the advantages of breast-feeding -- Checking out the benefits of bottle-feeding -- Latching onto breast-feeding -- Looking at the mechanics of lactation -- Checking out breast-feeding positions -- Getting the baby to latch on -- Orchestrating feedings -- Maintaining your diet -- Looking at birth control options -- Determining which medications are safe -- Handling common problems -- Breast-feeding twins -- Bottle-feeding for beginners -- Stopping milk production -- Choosing the best bottles and nipples -- Feeding your baby from a bottle -- Dealing with baby's developing digestive system. pt. IV. Dealing with special concerns -- 15. Pregnancies with special considerations -- Figuring out how age matters -- Over-30 something moms -- Not-so-young dads -- Very young moms --Having twins or more -- Looking at types of multiples -- Determining whether multiples are identical or fraternal -- Down syndrome screening in pregnancies with twins or more -- Genetic testing in pregnancies with twins or more -- Keeping track of which baby is which -- Living day-to-day during a multiple pregnancy -- Going through labor and delivery -- Covering special issues for moms with multiples -- Monitoring for preterm labor in twins -- Getting pregnant again -- Realizing how each pregnancy differs -- Giving birth after a prior cesarean delivery -- If you're a nontraditional family -- Preparing your child (or children) for a new arrival -- Explaining pregnancy -- Making baby-sitting arrangements for your delivery -- Coming home -- 16. When things get complicated -- Dealing with preterm labor -- Checking for signs of preterm labor -- Stopping preterm labor -- Preventing preterm labor -- Delivering the baby early -- Handling preeclampsia -- Understanding placental conditions -- Placenta previa -- Placental abruption -- Recognizing problems with the amniotic fluid and sac -- Too much amniotic fluid -- Too little amniotic fluid -- Rupture of the amniotic sac -- Describing problems with fetal growth -- Smaller-than-average babies -- Larger-than-average babies -- Looking at blood incompatibilities -- The Rh factor -- Other blood mismatches -- Dealing with breech presentation -- Pondering post-date pregnancy -- 17. Pregnancy in sickness and in health -- Getting an infection while pregnant -- Bladder and kidney infections -- Chickenpox -- Colds and flu -- Seasonal allergies and hay fever -- Cytomegalovirus (CMV) infections -- German measles (Rubella) -- Hepatitis -- Herpes infections -- Human immunodeficiency virus (HIV) -- Listeria -- Lyme disease -- Parvovirus infection (Fifth disease) -- Stomach viruses (gastroenteritis) -- Toxoplasmosis -- Vaginal infections -- Handling prepregnancy conditions -- Asthma -- Chronic hypertension -- Deep vein thrombosis and pulmonary embolus -- Diabetes -- Fibroids -- Immunological problems -- Inflammatory bowel disease -- Seizure disorders (epilepsy) -- Thyroid problems -- 18. Coping with the unexpected -- Surviving recurrent miscarriages -- Coping with late-pregnancy loss -- Dealing with fetal abnormalities -- Finding help -- Beginning to heal. pt. V. The part of tens -- 19. Ten things nobody tells you -- Pregnancy lasts longer than nine months -- Other people can drive you crazy -- You feel exhausted in the first trimester -- Round ligament pain really hurts -- Your belly becomes a hand magnet -- Hemorrhoids are a royal pain in the butt -- Sometimes women poop while pushing -- The weight stays on after the baby comes out -- Hospital pads are relics from your mother's era -- Breast engorgement really sucks and breast-feeding can be a production -- 20. Ten (or so) healthy snacks for pregnant women -- Chunky dried fig, coconut, and almond granola -- Guilt-free oatmeal cookies -- Peanut butter, chocolate, and banana quesadillas -- Double salmon dip -- Herbed cottage cheese dip with whole-grain bread -- Roasted tomatoes and mozzarella bites -- Chickpea parsley dip with pita chips and celery and carrot sticks -- Peanut butter and

	dried fruit bars -- Pregnancy for dummies fruit smoothie -- 21. Ten key things you can see on ultrasound -- Measurement of crown-rump length -- The face -- The spine -- The heart -- The hands -- The foot -- The fetal profile -- Three-dimensional image -- It's a boy! -- It's a girl! -- Index.
Subjects	Pregnancy--Popular works.
	Childbirth--Popular works.
Notes	Includes index.
Series	--For dummies

Prenatal and postnatal care: a woman-centered approach

LCCN	2013024996
Type of material	Book
Main title	Prenatal and postnatal care: a woman-centered approach / edited by Robin G. Jordan, Julie Marfell, Janet Engstrom, Cindy Farley.
Published/Produced	Ames, Iowa: Wiley-Blackwell, 2014.
Description	xxviii, 668 pages: illustrations; 28 cm.
ISBN	9780470960479 (paper: alk. paper)
	0470960477 (paper: alk. paper)
LC classification	RJ254 .P726 2014
Related names	Jordan, Robin G., 1954- editor of compilation.
	Marfell, Julie, editor of compilation.
	Engstrom, Janet, editor of compilation.
	Farley, Cindy L., editor of compilation.
Partial contents	pt. I. Physiological foundations of prenatal and postnatal care. 1. Reproductive tract structure and function / Patricia W. Caudle: Anatomy of the female reproductive system; Menstrual cycle physiology -- 2. Conception, implantation, and embryonic and fetal development / Patricia W. Caudle: Conception and implantation; The

placenta; The embryo; The fetus -- 3. Maternal physiological alterations during pregnancy / Patricia W. Caudle: Hematologic system adaptations; Cardiovascular changes; Respiratory adaptations; Renal adaptations; Gastrointestinal adaptations; Metabolic changes; Skin changes; Hair and nail changes; Immunologic changes; Neurological and sensory changes; Musculoskeletal adaptations; Endocrine changes -- pt. II. Preconception and prenatal care. 4. Preconception care / Victoria L. Baker: Challenges to providing preconception care; Benefits of preconception care; Evidence supporting preconception care; Content of preconception care -- 5. Prenatal care: goals, structure, and components / Carrie S. Klima: A brief history of prenatal care; Current goals for prenatal care; Structure of prenatal care; A new model of prenatal care: CenteringPregnancy; Components of prenatal care -- 6. Nutrition during pregnancy / Robin G. Jordan and Julie A. Paul: Understanding food units; Size of food servings; Prenatal nutrition and health outcomes; Nutritional needs in pregnancy; Macronutrients: total energy; Macronutrients: fats; Macronutrients: carbohydrates; Micronutrients; Weight gain in pregnancy; Food safety during pregnancy; Factors influencing nutritional intake; Making a nutritional assessment; Counseling for optimal prenatal nutrition; Special issues in nutrition -- 7. Pregnancy diagnosis and gestational age assessment / Janet L. Engstrom and Joyce D. Cappiello: Early pregnancy diagnosis and gestational age assessment; Pregnancy diagnosis; Gestational age assessment; Counseling for pregnancy diagnosis -- 8. Risk assessment and risk management in prenatal care / Robin G. Jordan: Process and purpose of risk assessment; Benefits of risk assessment; Limitations; Disadvantages of risk assessment and risk management; Misapplication of risk assessment and risk management; Perspective of risk and risk screening; Explaining risk to women; Potential problems of risk miscommunication; Informed consent -- 9. Prenatal genetic counseling, screening, and diagnosis / Robin G. Hordan and Janet L. Engstrom: Family history and risk evaluation; Genetic screening procedures offered to all pregnant women; Ethnicity-based genetic screening; Diagnostic prenatal genetic testing procedures; Developments in genetic testing options; Scope of practice considerations; Ethical considerations in genetic screening; Communicating about genetic testing and risk during prenatal care; Psychosocial effects in genetic testing; Perspective on genetic counseling during prenatal care -- 10. Assessment of fetal well-being / Jenifer Fahey: Physiological principles and indications for antenatal fetal surveillance; Scope of practice considerations; Antenatal fetal testing methods; Education and counseling; Cultural, personal, and family considerations; Health disparities and vulnerable populations; Legal and liability issues -- 11. Common disconforts of pregnancy / Robin G. Jordan: Back pain and pelvic girdle pain; Bleeding gums; Breast tenderness; Carpal tunnel syndrome (CTS); Cervical pain; Constipation; Dizziness/syncope; Edema; Emotional changes; Fatigue; Flatulence; Headache; Heartburn; Heart palpitations; Hemorrhoids; Increased warmth and perspiration; Leukorrhea; Leg cramps; Nasal congestion and epistaxis; Nausea and/or vomiting during pregnancy; Ptyalism; Restless leg syndrome (RLS); Round ligament pain; Shortness of breath; Skin changes; Hair and nail changes; Sleep disturbances; Supine hypotension syndrome (SHS); Urinary frequency; Urinary incontinence; Varicosities (legs/vulva); Visual changes -- 12. Medication use during pregnancy / Mary C. Brucker and Tekoa L. King: Pharmacologic terms; Types of pharmaceutical agents; Prescriptive authority; Governmental oversight of pharmaceutical agents; The prescription: essential components; Drugs and pregnancy; Teratology; Pharmacokinetics in pregnancy; Rational use of drugs in pregnancy -- 13. Substance use during pregnancy / Daisy J. Goodman, Alane B. O'Connor, and Kelley A. Bowden: Risks of perinatal substance abuse; Prevalence of prenatal substance abuse; Definitions; Historical approaches to maternal substance use; Harm reduction approach to prenatal substance abuse Position statements on prenatal substance use; Comorbid conditions and prenatal substance use; Commonly abused substances and pregnancy implications; Screening for prenatal substance abuse; Brief intervention and treatment; Smoking cessation during pregnancy; Care of pregnant women with substance use disorders; Referral to treatment; Opioid replacement therapy in pregnancy; Communication and coordination of care; Neonatal abstinence syndrome; Postpartum care; Cultural considerations; Personal and family considerations; Scope of practice considerations -- 14. Social issues in pregnancy / Nena R. Harris: Poverty; Incarceration; Intimate partner violence during pregnancy; Pregnancy and a history of childhood sexual abuse -- 15. Exercise, recreational and occupational issues, and intimate relationships in pregnancy / Meghan Garland: Exercise in pregnancy; Environmental exposures in pregnancy; Sexuality in pregnancy; Working during pregnancy -- 16. Psychosocial adaptations in pregnancy / Cindy L. Farley: Maternal attachment and adaptation; Sibling adaptation and attachment; Partner adaptation and attachment; Body image; Childbirth confidence -- 17. Health education during pregnancy / Lisa Hanson, Leona VandeVusse, and Kathryn Shisler Harrod: Sources and quality of consumer childbirth education; Prenatal visit approach to individual childbirth education; Class education and group prenatal care; Developmental considerations in prenatal health education; Issues integral to prenatal education; Prioritizing prenatal education needs; Trimester-based approaches to prenatal education; Cultural considerations; Health disparities and vulnerable populations;

Documentation of teaching -- 18. Assessment and care at the onset of labor / Amy Marowitz: Determining the onset of labor; Timing of admission to the birth setting; What is "false labor"?; Determining active labor; Anticipatory guidance during the prenatal period; Data collection; Plan of care; Sleep and rest; Coping strategies and comfort measures for early labor; Ambulation in early labor -- pt. III. Common complications of pregnancy. 19. Bleeding during pregnancy / Robin G. Jordan: Bleeding during the first half of pregnancy; Evaluation; Subchorionic hemorrhage or hematoma; Leiomyomas; Spontaneous pregnancy loss; Ectopic pregnancy; Gestational trophoblastic disease; Early pregnancy bleeding and scope of practice considerations; Bleeding during the second half of pregnancy; Placenta previa; Placental abruption; Diagnosis and management of bleeding in the second half of pregnancy; Scope of practice considerations in later pregnancy bleeding; Family considerations in later pregnancy -- 20. Amniotic fluid and fetal growth disorders / Victoria H. Burslem and Cindy L. Farley: Amniotic fluid dynamics; Normal placentation and fetal development; Amniotic fluid disorders; Fetal growth disorders; Intrauterine growth restriction -- 21. Preterm labor and birth / Robin G. Jordan: Social and racial disparities; Physiology of preterm birth; Complications related to prematurity; Risk factors for preterm birth; Predicting preterm birth; Diagnosing preterm birth; Management of women with preterm labor; Preterm birth prevention; Progesterone therapy; Cerclage -- 22. Hypertensive disorders in pregnancy / Robin G. Jordan: Classification of hypertensive disorders of pregnancy; Chronic hypertension; Gestational hypertension; Preeclampsia-eclampsia; Preeclampsia superimposed on chronic hypertension; Preeclampsia; HELLP syndrome; Atypical presentation preeclampsia; Prediction of preeclampsia; Prevention of preeclampsia; Long-term sequelae of preeclampsia; Risk management issues in the office setting; Interprofessional practice issues -- 23. Gestational diabetes / Kimberly K. Trout: Pathophysiology and potential problems of gestational diabetes; Prenatal screening and diagnosis of GDM; Management of gestational diabetes; Oral medications for GDM; Insulin therapy; Fetal surveillance and timing of birth; Postpartum follow-up; Scope of practice issues; Perspective on GDM risk -- 24. Other complications in pregnancy: multiple gestation, post-term pregnancy, hyperemesis, and abdominal pain / Tonya B. Nicholson: Abdominal pain in pregnancy; Hyperemesis gravidarum (HG); Multifetal pregnancy; Post-term pregnancy -- 25. Perinatal loss and grief / Robin G. Jordan: Stillbirth; Breaking the news; Care and management of women with stillbirth; Grieving and emotional care after perinatal loss; Physical care after stillbirth; Follow-up; Interconception and subsequent pregnancy care -- pt. IV. Postnatal care. 26. Physiological alterations during the postnatal period /

Kimberly A. Couch and Karen DeCocker-Geist: Uterus; Lochia; Cervix; Vagina; Labia and perineum; Additional maternal alterations during the postpartum period -- 27. Components of postnatal care / Tia P. Andrighetti and Deborah Brandt Karsnitz: Assessment of maternal physical and emotional adjustment; Activity/exercise; Diet and nutrition; Lochia; Afterbirth pain; Perineal discomfort; Diureseis/diaphoresis; Constipation/hemorrhoids; Sexuality; Resumption of menses and ovulation; Contraception; Postpartum physical examination; Postpartum depression and domestic violence screening; Postnatal warning signs; Cultural considerations; Health disparities and vulnerable populations; Scope of practice considerations; Legal issues -- 28. Common complications during the postnatal period / Deborah Brandt Karsnitz: Postpartum morbidity and mortality; Postpartum cultural considerations; Postpartum disorders -- 29. Contraception / Patricia Aikins Murphy and Leah N. Torres: Postpartum care and return to fertility after childbirth; Considerations in selecting a postpartum contraceptive method; Contraceptive methods; Tier one methods; Tier two methods; Tier three methods; Emergency contraception -- 30. Lactation and breastfeeding / Marsha Walker: Breastfeeding as a public health issue; The unique properties of human milk; Nutritional properties of human milk; Maternal and infant anatomy and physiology of lactation and breastfeeding; Promoting and supporting breastfeeding; The basics of breastfeeding support and assessment; Milk production; Breastfeeding patterns; Assessing intake; Care of the breastfeeding mother -- 31. Common breastfeeding problems / Marsha Walker: Common infant-related breastfeeding problems; Common maternal breastfeeding problems; Breast engorgement; Mastitis; Abscess; Low milk supply -- pt. V. Management of common health problems during the prenatal and postnatal periods. 32. Respiratory disorders / Janyce Cagan Agruss: Respiratory physiology and pregnancy; Asthma; Influenza; Upper respiratory infection; Pneumonia -- 33. Hematological and thromboembolic disorders / Julie A. Marfell: Anemia; Iron-deficiency anemia; Hemoglobinopathies; Folate deficiency; Vitamin B&#27;b12&#27;s deficiency; Unexplained maternal anemia; Bleeding disorders; Coagulopathies during pregnancy -- 34. Urinary tract disorders / Rhonda Arthur and Nancy Pesta Walsh: Urinary tract infection; Evaluation; Care of women with urinary tract infections; Recurrent UTI; Care of women with suspected acute pyelonephritis; Nephrolithiasis -- 35. Gastrointestinal disorders / Audra C. Malone and Karen DeCocker-Geist: Gastroenteritis; Intraheptic cholestasis of pregnancy; Cholecystitis; Appendicitis -- 36. Obesity / Cecelia M. Jevitt: Overview; Prevalence; Health disparities and cultural considerations; Personal and family considerations; Obesity physiology; Potential problems associated with obesity in childbearing women; Management of pregestational obesity; Management principles; Nutrition; Weight loss concerns; Physical activity; Comfort measures; Bariatric surgery; Scope of practice considerations; Legal and liability issues; Intrapartum and postpartum issues -- 37. Endocrine disorders / Elizabeth Gabzdyl: Thyroid disorders in pregnancy; Diagnosing thyroid disorders; Overt hypothyroidism; Subclinical hypothyroidism; Screening for hypothyroidism in pregnancy; Preconception care of a woman with hypothyroidism; Hyperthyroidism; Subclinical hyperthyroidism; Thyroid storm; Postpartum thyroiditis; Pregestational diabetes -- 38. Neurological disorders / Tonya B. Nicholson: Care of the pregnant woman; Care of pregnant women with headacle; Care of pregnant women with multiple sclerosis -- 39. Dermatological disorders / Gwendolyn Short and Elizabeth Powell Holcomb: Atopic dermatitis; Prurigo of pregnancy; Pruritic urticarial papules and plaques of pregnancy; Pruritic folliculitis of pregnancy; Pemphigoid gestationis; Impetigo herpetiformis; Intrahepatic cholestasis of pregnancy -- 40. Infectious diseases / Jacquelyne Brooks and Elizabeth A. Parr: Cytomegalovirus; Group B streptococcus; Hepatitis infections; Parvovirus B19; Rubella; Toxoplasmosis; Varicella -- 41. Sexually transmitted infections and common vaginitis / Meghan Garland and Barbara P. Brennan: Sexually transmitted bacterial infections;

	Sexually transmitted viral infections; Fungal infection; Sexually transmitted parasitic infection; Sexually transmitted bacterial infection; Partner treatment of an STI; Legal requirements for reporting STI diagnosis; Psychosocial impacts of STI diagnosis -- 42. Psychological disorders / Heather Shlosser: Overview; Depression during pregnancy; Bipolar disorder in pregnancy; Generalized anxiety disorder (GAD); Scope of practice considerations.
Subjects	Neonatal nursing.
	Neonatal Nursing.
	Patient-Centered Care.
	Pregnancy--physiology.
	Pregnancy Complications--nursing.
	Women's Health.
Notes	Includes bibliographical references and index.

Qualitative research in midwifery and childbirth phenomenological approaches

LCCN	2010049023
Type of material	Book
Main title	Qualitative research in midwifery and childbirth phenomenological approaches / edited by Gill Thomson, Fiona Dykes, and Soo Downe.
Edition	First edition.
Published/Created	London; New York: Routledge, 2011.
Description	xix, 244 p.: ill.; 25 cm.
ISBN	9780415575010 (hbk)
	9780203816820 (ebk)
LC classification	RG950 .Q35 2011
Related names	Thomson, Gill, editor.
	Dykes, Fiona, editor.

Contents

Downe, Soo, editor.
Husserlian phenomenology reflected in caring science childbearing research / Terese Bondas -- Lifeworld phenomenology for caring and health care research / Karin Dahlberg -- From beginning to end: how to do hermeneutic interpretive phenomenology / Elizabeth Smythe -- Phenomenological research approaches: mapping the terrain of competing perspectives / Maura Dowling -- Lesbian women's experiences of being different in Irish health care / Mel Duffy -- Women's lived experiences of severe early onset of preeclampsia: a hermeneutic analysis / Joyce Cowan, Elizabeth Smythe & Marion Hunter -- The meaning of giving birth from a long-term perspective for childbearing women / Ingela Lundgren -- Abandonment of being in childbirth / Gill Thomson -- Parents' participation in the care of their child in neonatal intensive care / Marie Berg & Helena Wigert -- A poetic hermeneutic phenomenological analysis of midwives being with woman during childbirth / Lauren Hunter -- Revealing the subtle differences among postpartum mood and anxiety disorders: phenomenology holds the key / Cheryl Tatano Beck -- Heidegger's contribution to hermeneutic phenomenological research / Maria Healy -- Authenticity and poetics: what is different about phenomenology / Soo Downe, Gill Thomson & Fiona Dykes.

Subjects

Midwifery--Research--Methodology.
Qualitative research.
Parturition.

	Midwifery.
	Philosophy.
	Postnatal Care.
	Postpartum Period--psychology.
	Qualitative Research.
Notes	Includes bibliographical references and index.

Rapid review anesthesiology oral boards

LCCN	2013020827
Type of material	Book
Main title	Rapid review anesthesiology oral boards / edited by Ruchir Gupta; associate editor, Minh Chau Joseph Tran.
Published/Produced	Cambridge: Cambridge University Press, 2013.
Description	xx, 239 pages; 24 cm.
ISBN	9781107653665 (pbk.: alk. paper)
LC classification	RD82.3 .R37 2013
Related names	Gupta, Ruchir, editor of compilation.
	Tran, Minh Chau Joseph, editor of compilation.
Summary	"Written for trainees who are preparing to take the Anesthesia Oral Board exam, Rapid Review Anesthesiology Oral Boards is focused on the most commonly tested topics on the ABA oral board exam. Presented in a question-and-answer format, the book covers 39 different clinical scenarios encountered in the exam, including the Parkland formula to calculate fluid resuscitation in burn patients, ICP monitoring in craniotomy and hemodynamic goals in patients with cardiac disease. Questions follow the normal course of a case, from pre-operative assessment to intra-operative management and post-operative care. The answers to the questions are carefully structured to not only

Bibliography

Contents

help the reader understand the medicine of anesthesia but also to provide the correct terminology needed to successfully pass the exam. This book is essential reading for trainees preparing for one of the toughest exams of their careers"--Provided by publisher.

Introduction; Part I. General: 1. Obesity/difficult airway / Ruchir Gupta -- 2. Myasthenia gravis/Eaton-Lambert syndrome / Shimon Frankel -- 3. Laryngeal papillomatosis / Aimee Gretchen Kakascik -- 4. Sickle cell disease / Ruchir Gupta -- 5. Liver transplant / Federico Osorio -- 6. Renal transplant/diabetes / Ruchir Gupta, Anita Gupta and Sheryl Glassman. Part II. Endocrine: 7. Thyroidectomy / Ruchir Gupta -- 8. Carcinoid tumor / Xiaodong Bao -- 9. Pheochromocytoma / Stanley Yuan and John Cooley. Part III. Orthopedics: 10. Shoulder surgery / Sarah J. Madison; 11. Hip replacement in aortic stenosis Ruchir Gupta; Part IV. Trauma: 12. The burn patient Ruchir Gupta; 13. Multisystem injury Raymond Pesso -- 14. Traumatic brain injury / Ruchir Gupta. Part V. Urology: 15. TURP syndrome / Mark Slomovits. Part VI. Pediatrics: 16. Foreign body aspiration / Aimee Gretchen Kakascik -- 17. Tracheoesophageal fistula repair / Peggy Wingard -- 18. Pyloric stenosis / Julio R. Olaya -- 19. Congenital diaphragmatic hernia / Peggy Wingard -- 20. Epiglottitis / Julio R. Olaya -- 21. Patent ductus arteriosis / Peggy Wingard -- 22. Tetralogy of fallout Ruchir Gupta. Part VII. Neuro: 23. Intracranial mass / Sergey V. Pisklakov -- 24. Cerebral aneurysm / Sergey V.

	Pisklakov. Part VIII. Thoracic: 25. VATS (one-lung ventilation) / Ruchir Gupta -- 26. Mediastinal mass Stanley Yuan and Joseph Marino. Part IX. Cardiovascular: 27. Aortic dissection / Ruchir Gupta -- 28. Carotid endarterectomy / Ruchir Gupta -- 29. Coronary artery bypass graft (CABG) / Ruchir Gupta -- 30. Abdominal aortic aneurysm / Ruchir Gupta -- Part X. Obstetric: 31. Hemorrhage / Edouard Belotte -- 32. Preeclampsia / Xiaodong Bao. Part XI. Additional Topics: 33. Cardiac / Ruchir Gupta -- 34. Obstetrics / Anita Gupta and Nicholas Weber -- 35. Pediatrics / Ruchir Gupta, Monique Cadogan and Barbara Vickers -- 36. Neuro / Ruchir Gupta -- 37. Pain management / Ruchir Gupta -- 38. Neuraxial anesthesia/anticoagulation / Ruchir Gupta -- 39. Critical care / Ruchir Gupta.
Subjects	Anesthesiology--methods--Examination Questions.
	Anesthesia--Examination Questions.
	Anesthetics--Examination Questions.
Notes	Includes bibliographical references and index.

Real nursing simulations facilitator's guide: institutional version

LCCN	2008022396
Type of material	Book
Main title	Real nursing simulations facilitator's guide: institutional version
Published/Created	Upper Saddle River, NJ: Pearson Prentice Hall, c2009.
Description	xxi, 281 p.: ill.; 28 cm.
Links	Table of contents only http://www.loc.gov/catdir/toc/ecip0819/2008022396.html

ISBN	9780135042489
	0135042488
LC classification	RT81.6 .R388 2009
Related names	Pearson/Prentice Hall.
Contents	Well child 6-month visit (Jamie Tyler) -- Septic shock (Jethro Land) -- Infant non-accidental trauma (Julia Faslon) -- Surgical consent for client in pain (Jason Plaxx) -- Sickle cell crisis (Michael Mason) -- Diabetic ketoacidosis (DKA), type 1 diabetes mellitus (Norma Gaul) -- Hemorrhagic shock (Jane Souza) -- Postoperative care, ulcerative colitis requiring ileostomy (Carmela Lewis) -- Primary hypertension (James Wilson) -- Type 2 diabetes (Jack Taylor) -- Chronic obstructive pulmonary disease (COPD) (Cindy Lui) -- Congestive heart failure (Helen Martinez) -- Upper respiratory infection with asthma (Raven McDonald) -- Hyperkalemia (Hiram Winston) -- Preeclampsia (Shantell Gaines) -- Adolescent depression (Amy Beckman) -- Postoperative pneumonia (Hal Trand) -- Respiratory distress (Juan Sanchez-Ramirez) -- Acute pain (Lucille Larson) -- Acute renal failure (Lucille Larson) -- End of life care (Lucille Larson).
Subjects	Nursing--Case studies.
	Nursing Care--Case Reports.

SOAP for obstetrics and gynecology

LCCN	2004005831
Type of material	Book
Personal name	Uzelac, Peter S.
Main title	SOAP for obstetrics and gynecology / Peter S. Uzelac.

Published/Created	Malden, Mass.: Blackwell Pub., c2005.
Description	xx, 143 p.; 22 cm.
Links	Book review (E-STREAMS) http://www.e-streams.com/es0803/es0803_3994.html
	Publisher description http://www.loc.gov/catdir/enhancements/fy0712/2004005831-d.html
ISBN	140510435X (pbk.)
LC classification	RG110 .U985 2005
Contents	Initial visit -- Second trimester visit -- Third trimester visit -- Postpartum visit -- Anemia -- Antiphospholipid syndrome -- Asthma -- Chronic hypertension -- Gestational diabetes -- Hyperthyroidism -- Intrauterine growth restriction -- Isoimmunization -- Mild preeclampsia -- Nausea and vomiting of pregnancy -- Seizure disorder -- Severe preeclampsia -- Systemic lupus erythematosus -- Twin gestation -- Urinary tract infection -- Term labor -- Third trimester bleeding -- Chorioamnionitis -- Labor dystocia -- Preterm labor -- Pyelonephritis -- Rupture of membranes -- Postpartum day 1 -- Postpartum day 2 -- Dyspnea -- Postpartum fever -- Postpartum hemorrhage -- Well woman exam -- Abnormal uterine bleeding -- Breast mass -- Chronic pelvic pain -- Dysmenorrhea -- Family planning-barrier method -- Family planning-depot mpa -- Family planning-emergency contraception -- Family planning-intrauterine device -- Family planning-oral contraceptives -- Family planning-sterilization -- Galactorrhea -- Hirsutism -- Infertility -- Menopause -- Perimenopause -- Premenstrual syndrome -- Recurrent pregnancy loss -- Secondary

	amenorrhea -- Std screening -- Urinary incontinence -- Vulvar ulcers -- Vulvovaginitis -- First trimester bleeding-abortion -- First trimester bleeding-ectopic pregnancy -- Acute pelvic pain -- Gestational trophoblastic disease -- Pelvic inflammatory disease -- Pelvic mass -- Postoperative day 1 -- Postoperative day 2 -- Postoperative days 3 and 4.
Subjects	Obstetrics--Handbooks, manuals, etc. Gynecology--Handbooks, manuals, etc. Genital Diseases, Female--Handbooks. Obstetrics--Handbooks. Pregnancy Complications--Handbooks.
Notes	Includes index.
Series	SOAP series

The everything guide to pregnancy over 35: from conquering your fears to assessing health risks--all you need to have a happy, healthy nine months

LCCN	2007015890
Type of material	Book
Personal name	Sember, Brette McWhorter.
Main title	The everything guide to pregnancy over 35: from conquering your fears to assessing health risks--all you need to have a happy, healthy nine months / Brette McWhorter Sember; technical review by Bruce D. Rodgers and Diane E. Rodgers.
Published/Created	Avon, Mass.: Adams Media, c2007.
Description	xii, 289 p.; 24 cm.
ISBN	9781598692457 (pbk.) 1598692453 (pbk.)
LC classification	RG556.6 .S46 2007
Variant title	Everything guide to pregnancy over thirty-five

	Guide to pregnancy over thirty-five
	Pregnancy over thirty-five
Portion of title	Guide to pregnancy over 35
	Pregnancy over 35
Related names	Rodgers, Bruce D.
	Rodgers, Diane E.
Summary	Discusses the physical, social, and emotionals implications of midlife motherhood, covering such topics as proper nutrition, the benefits and risks of prenatal testing, and financial and career considerations.
Contents	Top ten reasons to have a baby after age 35 -- Introduction -- 1. Deciding to become a parent -- Evaluating if you want a child -- Making room in your life for a child -- Impact on you r career -- Impact on your relationships -- Impact on your finances -- Benefits of being a mom over 35 -- 2. Avenues to parenthood -- Single moms -- Adoption -- Blended families -- Same-sex couples -- Unplanned pregnancy -- Pregnancy after loss -- Facing pregnancy again -- 3. Fertility -- Your biological clock -- Finding a specialist -- Determining if there is a problem -- Fertility tests -- Fertility drugs -- Insemination -- In-vitro fertilization (IVF) -- Surrogacy -- New options - Staying sane through fertility treatments -- 4. Preconception planning -- Checkup -- Vitamins -- Drugs and pre-existing conditions -- What to avoid -- Starting at a healthy weight -- Exercise -- Genetic counseling -- Understanding your cycle -- Your partner's health -- 5. Staying healthy during pregnancy -- Weight gain and nutrition -- Exercise -- nausea -- Sleep difficulties -- Aches and pains --

Emotional ups and downs -- 6. How an over-35 pregnancy is managed -- Deciding on a health-care provider -- Finding a health-care provider -- Planning your medical care -- Asking questions and educating yourself -- Taking control of your own health care -- How an over-35 pregnancy is monitored -- Your birth plan -- 7. Risks -- Calming your fears and understanding risks -- Reducing risks -- Gestational diabetes -- Preeclampsia -- Placenta previa -- Low birth weight -- Preterm birth -- Multiples -- Birth defects -- 8. Prenatal testing -- How to think about and approach testing -- Ultrasounds -- Blood tests -- Combination tests -- Fundal height -- Genetic counseling -- Chorionic villus sampling (CVS) -- Amniocentesis -- Nonstress test -- 9. Pregnancy loss -- Miscarriage -- Ectopic pregnancy -- Stillbirth -- Multifetal pregnancy reduction -- Pregnancy termination -- Recovering from loss -- Trying again -- 10. preparing your family for a baby -- Work leaves and career changes -- Other children -- Lifestyle changes -- Classes -- Planning for the future -- Preparing your home -- Making plans for help -- 11. Protecting your family -- Financial planning -- Health insurance and medical savings accounts -- Wills -- Health-care directives -- Life insurance -- College savings -- Cord blood preservation -- 12. Feeling good throughout your pregnancy -- Managing stress -- Dealing with worries and fears -- Sex and intimacy -- Coping with pregnancy problems -- Finding support -- Working while pregnant -- 13. Loving your pregnant self -- Dealing with body changes -- Accepting that you must do less -- Changing your perception of who you are -- Listening to your body -- Not letting pregnancy take over you life -- Dressing the part -- 15. Labor and delivery -- The role of your coach -- Choosing a birth facility -- Pain-relief options -- Labor induction and augmentation -- Vaginal birth -- Vaginal birth after Cesarean (VBAC) -- Alternatives to traditional hospital birth -- 16. Cesarean sections (C-sections) -- C-section basics -- Reasons for C-sections -- How to decrease your chances -- What to expect -- Pain relief -- 17. Recovery -- Recovery from vaginal birth -- Recovery from C-section -- Postpartum depression -- Coping with sleep deprivation -- Nursing or bottlefeeding -- Discovering yourself as a mother -- Your relationship as parents -- Weight loss -- 18. Working and parenting -- Deciding when to return to work -- Day care -- Relative care -- Hiring a nanny -- Changing your schedule -- Working at home -- Becoming an at-home mom -- Sharing the parenting burden -- 19. Life as an older mom -- Enjoying every moment -- Readjusting priorities and expectations -- Sandwich generation -- Finding time for you -- Finding time for your partner -- Finding time for your other children -- Finding support -- 20. Your health after pregnancy -- Birth control -- Menopause -- Estrogen replacement -- Health risks as you age -- Getting pregnant again -- Appendix A: Helpful web sites -- Appendix B: Additional resources -- Index.

Subjects	Pregnancy in middle age--Popular works.
	Childbirth in middle age--Popular works.
Notes	Includes bibliographical references (p. 275-279) and index.
Series	The everything series

The long term impact of medical complications in pregnancy: a window into maternal and fetal future health

LCCN	2016027862
Type of material	Book
Main title	The long term impact of medical complications in pregnancy: a window into maternal and fetal future health / edited by Eyal Sheiner, MD, PhD, Professor and Chairman, Department of Obstetrics and Gynecology B, Soroka University Medical Center, and Vice Dean, Student Affairs, Faculty of Health Sciences, Ben-Gurion University of the Negev, Be'er Sheva, Israel.
Published/Produced	Boca Raton: CRC Press, Taylor & Francis Group, 2017.
Description	xiii, 242 pages: illustrations; 25 cm.
ISBN	9781498764674 (pbk.)
	1498764673 (pbk.)
LC classification	RG571 .L66 2017
Related names	Sheiner, Eyal, editor.
Contents	Preeclampsia and long-term maternal atherosclerotic and cardiovascular disease / Yoav Yinon -- Gestational diabetes mellitus: definition, pregnancy complications, and long-term maternal complications / Shelly Meshel and Yariv Yogev -- Placental syndrome and long-term maternal complications / Gali Pariente, Tom Leibson, Howard Berger, and

Eyal Sheiner -- Pregnancy complications and long-term oncological morbidity of the mother / Roy Kessous and Walter H Gotlieb -- Recurrent pregnancy loss: overview and impact on future maternal health / Oren Barak and Edi Vaisbuch -- Preterm parturition and long term maternal morbidity / Salvatore Andrea Mastrolia, Shirley Greenbaum, Vered Klaitman, Ruthy Beer-Weisel, Shiran Zer, Gal Rodavsky, Idit Erez-Weiss, and Offer Erez -- Renal function tests during pregnancy and long-term risk for maternal therosclerotic morbidity / Leah Shalev and Talya Wolak -- Pregnancy and depression: the tip of the iceberg? / Samantha Meltzer-Brody -- Pregnancy and thromboembolic morbidity / Zeva Daniela Herzog Aaron Herzog, and Eyal Sheiner -- Cholestasis and long-term maternal morbidity / Hans-Ulrich Marschall -- Fertility treatment and maternal cardiovascular risk / Judah Weiss and Avi Harlev -- Pregnancy as an opportunity for weight-control and smoking cessation / Asnat Walfisch -- Preeclampsia and long-term risk for the offspring / Kira Sacks and Eyal Sheiner -- Life-course outcomes for the child of the diabetic mother / Jonah Susser Kreniske, Ron Charach, and Eyal Sheiner -- Intrauterine growth restriction and long term disease of the offspring / Tal Biron-Shental and Hannah Glinter -- Long-term effects of premature birth / Grace Eunjin Lee and Kent Willis -- The long-term health outcomes for children born as a result of in vitro fertilization treatment / Jennifer Mary Alice Beale, Jennifer Claire Pontré, and

	Roger Hart -- Long term impact of antidepressant exposure in pregnancy: a window into developmental outcomes in the child / Salvatore Gentile.
Subjects	Pregnancy Complications
	Maternal Health
	Infant Health
	Pregnancy Outcome
Notes	Includes bibliographical references and index.
Series	Series in maternal-fetal medicine, 2158-0855
	Series in maternal-fetal medicine. 2158-0855

The natural way to a trouble-free pregnancy: the toxemia-thiamine connection

LCCN	2008008530
Type of material	Book
Personal name	Irwin, John B.
Main title	The natural way to a trouble-free pregnancy: the toxemia-thiamine connection / by John B. Irwin.
Published/Created	Fairfield, CT.: Aslan Pub., c2008.
Description	xvi, 192 p.; 24 cm.
Links	Table of contents only http://www.loc.gov/cat dir/toc/ecip0812/2008008530.html
ISBN	9780944031780 (alk. paper)
	0944031781 (alk. paper)
LC classification	RG575 .I79 2008
Summary	"Simple explanations for pregnant women about why and how to take high-dose thiamine [vitamin B1]. Women can inexpensively and safely prevent toxemia and prematurity. Natural megathiamine prevented toxemia completely in over 1,000 pregnancies in hospitals in USA, Saipan, and Australia. No maternal or fetal

	deaths, no prematurity, no hemorrhaging, no hypertension, no preeclampsia, and no side reactions"--Provided by publisher.
Subjects	Toxemia of pregnancy.
	Vitamin B1--Therapeutic use.
	Pregnancy--Complications.
Notes	Includes bibliographical references (p. 167-169) and index.

Vitamin E and health

LCCN	2004028983
Type of material	Book
Main title	Vitamin E and health / edited by Frank Kelly, Mohsen Meydani, and Lester Packer.
Published/Created	New York, N.Y.: New York Academy of Sciences, 2004.
Description	xiii, 463 p.: ill.; 23 cm.
Links	Table of contents http://www.loc.gov/catdir/toc/ecip054/2004028983.html
ISBN	1573315273 (cloth: alk. paper)
	1573315281 (pbk.: alk. paper)
LC classification	Q11 .N5 vol. 1031 QP772.T6
Related names	Kelly, Frank J.
	Meydani, Mohsen.
	Packer, Lester.
Contents	Vitamin E trafficking / by Maret G. Traber, Graham W. Burton, and Robert L. Hamilton -- Discovery, characterization, and significance of the cytochrome P450 v-hydroxylase pathway of vitamin E catabolism / by Robert S. Parker ... [et al.] -- Inter- and intra-individual vitamin E uptake in healthy subjects is highly repeatable across a wide supplementation dose range / by Frank J. Kelly, Rosalind Le, and Ian S. Mudway

-- The effect of age on vitamin E status, metabolism, and function metabolism as assessed by labeled tocopherols / by Regina Brigelius-Flohé ... [et al.] -- Molecular mechanisms of vitamin E transport / by Achim Stocker -- Physiological factors influencing vitamin E biokinetics / by John K. Lodge ... [et al.] -- A-tocopherol and endothelial nitric oxide synthesis / by Regine Heller, Gabriele Werner-Felmayer, and Ernst R. Werner -- Vitamin E mediates cell signaling and regulation of gene expression / Angelo Azzi ... [et al.] -- Vitamin E and gene expression in immune cells / by Sung Nim Han ... [et al.] -- Modulation of hepatic gene expression by A-tocopherol in cultured cells and in vivo / by Gerald Rimbach ... [et al.] -- A-tocopherol transfer protein deficiency in mice causes multi-organ deregulation of gene networks and behavioral deficits with age / by Kishorchandra Gohil ... [et al.] -- Tocotrienol: the natural vitamin E to defend the nervous system? / by Chandan K. Sen, Savita Khanna, and Sashwati Roy -- Tocotrienol-rich fraction from palm oil and gene expression in human breast cancer cells / by Kalanithi Nesaretnam ... [et al.] -- Vitamin E and the oxidative stress of exercise / by M.J. Jackson ... [et al.] -- Effect of vitamin E on gene expression changes in diet-related carcinogenesis / by Joseph Lunec ...[et al.] -- Oral supplementation with ALL-RAR- and RRR-A-tocopherol increases vitamin E levels in human sebum after a latency period of 14-21 days / by Swarna Ekanayake-Mudiyanselage, Klaus Kraemer, and Jens J.

	Thiele -- Anti-inflammatory effects of A-tocopherol / by Uma Singh and Ishwarlal Jialal -- Oxidative stress and antioxidant treatment in diabetes / by Joshua A. Scott and George L. King -- Vitamin E and respiratory infection in the elderly / by Simin Nikbin Meydani, Sung Nim Han, and Davidson H. Hamer -- Tocopherols and the treatment of colon cancer / By William L. Stone ... [et al.] -- Selenium and vitamin E cancer prevention trial / by Eric A. Klein -- Vitamin E in preeclampsia / by Lucilla Poston, Maarten Raijmakers, and Frank Kelly -- Vitamin E in neurodegenerative disorders: Alzheimer's disease / by Anatol Kontush and Svetlana Schekatolina -- Vitamin E in neural and visual function / by S.M. Hayton AND D.P.R. Muller -- Vitamin E modulation of cardiovascular disease / by Mohsen Meydani -- Vitamin E and cardiovascular disease: observational studies / by J. Michael Gaziano -- Vitamin E for the treatment of cardiovascular disease: is there a future? / by Francesco Violi ... [et al.] -- Short papers.
Subjects	Vitamin E--Health aspects--Congresses.
	Vitamin E--physiology--Congresses.
	Vitamin E--therapeutic use--Congresses.
Notes	Based on a conference held May 22-24, 2004, in Boston, Mass.
	Includes bibliographical references and index.
Series	Annals of the New York Academy of Sciences; v. 1031

Williams manual of pregnancy complications
LCCN   2012026521

Type of material	Book
Main title	Williams manual of pregnancy complications / senior editor, Kenneth J. Leveno; associate editors, James M. Alexander ... [et al.].
Edition	23rd ed.
Published/Created	New York: McGraw-Hill Professional, c2013.
ISBN	9780071765626 (alk. paper)
Variant title	Manual of pregnancy compliations
Related titles	William's manual of obstetrics. Williams obstetrics.
Related names	Leveno, Kenneth J. Alexander, James M., 1965-
Summary	"The only pocket manual derived from Williams Obstetrics, 23e -- completely updated and now in full color Williams Manual of Pregnancy Complications, 23e is a carry-anywhere, condensed guide to the Williams protocols for diagnosis and management of complications and illnesses during pregnancy. Reflecting the rigorously referenced, evidence-based approach of the parent text, the manual delivers essential information on: Prenatal screening Mediation use in pregnancy Hypertension disorders in pregnancy Pain management dosages Procedures for complicated labor and delivery, hemoglobinopathies, and more Thoroughly cross-referenced to Williams Obstetrics, 23e for the latest literature citations, this edition is enhanced by a new full-color presentation, more tables and algorithms, and an increased emphasis on diagnosis and treatment. There is no faster or more efficient way to access the key facts, diagnostic tools, and treatment guidelines

found in Williams Obstetrics, 23e than this authoritative, streamlined sourcebook"-- Provided by publisher.

Contents

Machine generated contents note: Part I: Obstetrical Complications due to Pregnancy 1. Early Pregnancy Loss 2. Ectopic Pregnancy 3. Screening for Neural-Tube Defects, Down Syndrome, and Heritable Genetic Diseases 4. Prenatal Diagnosis 5. Chromosomal Abnormalities 6. Single-Gene (Mendelian) Disorders 7. Nonmendelian Disorders 8. Teratology, Medications, and Substance Abuse 9. Ultrasound Imaging Including Doppler Velocimetry 10. Oligohydramnios 11. Hydramnios 12. Antepartum Fetal Testing 13. Intrapartum Fetal Heart Rate Assessment 14. Abnormal Labor and Delivery 15. Chorioamnionitis 16. Shoulder Dystocia 17. Breech Delivery 18. Prior Cesarean Delivery 19. Uterine Rupture 20. Hysterectomy Following Delivery 21. Postpartum and Postoperative Infections 22. Septic Pelvic Thrombophlebitis 23. Gestational Hypertension and Preeclampsia 24. Eclampsia 25. Placental Abruption 26. Placenta Previa 27. Fetal-to-Maternal Hemorrhage 28. Hemorrhage Immediately Following Delivery 29. Transfusion of Blood Products for Obstetrical Hemorrhage 30. Amnionic Fluid Embolism 31. Fetal Death and Delayed Delivery 32. Preterm Birth: Definitions, Consequences, and Causes 33. Prediction of Preterm Birth 34. Preterm Ruptured Membranes 35. Preterm Birth: Intact Membranes 36. Incompetent Cervix 37.

Postterm Pregnancy 38. Fetal Growth Restriction 39. Macrosomia 40. Twin Pregnancy: Overview 41. Complications Unique to Twins 42. Triplets and More 43. Selective Reduction or Termination of Multifetal Pregnancy 44. Gestational Trophoblastic Disease Part II: Medical and Surgical Complications during Pregnancy 45. Active Pulmonary Edema and Adult Respiratory Distress Syndrome 46. Pulmonary Artery Catheterization 47. Chronic Hypertension 48. Heart Disease in Pregnancy 49. Pneumonia 50. Asthma 51. Tuberculosis, Sarcoid and Cystic Fibrosis 52. Thromboembolic Disease 53. Thrombophilias 54. Antiphospholipid Antibody Syndrome 55. Systemic Lupus Erythematosus 56. Rheumatoid Arthritis and Other Connective-Tissue Disorders 57. Hyperemesis Gravidarum 58. Cholestasis of Pregnancy 59. Diseases of the Gallbladder and Pancreas 60. Appendicitis 61. Viral Hepatitis 62. Acute Fatty Liver of Pregnancy 63. Asymptomatic Bacteriuria (ASB) 64. Cystitis 65. Acute Pyelonephritis 66. Nephrolithiasis 67. Acute and Chronic Renal Failure 68. Anemia 69. Hemoglobinopathies 70. Thrombocytopenia 71. Gestational Diabetes 72. Pregestational Overt Diabetes 73. Hypothyroidism 74. Hyperthyroidism 75. Postpartum Thyroiditis 76. Epilepsy 77. Cerebrovascular Diseases 78. Other Neurologic Disorders 79. Psychiatric Illnesses During Pregnancy 80. Postpartum Depression 81. Cancer During Pregnancy 82. Dermatological

Bibliography 163

	Disorders 83. Sexually Transmitted Diseases 84. Group A and B Streptococcus Infections 85. Human Immunodeficiency Virus 86. Cytomegalovirus, Parvovirus, Varicella, Rubella, Toxoplasmosis, Listeria, and Malaria 87. Trauma in Pregnancy 88. Surgery During Pregnancy Part III: Complications in the Fetus or Newborn Infant 89. Resuscitation of the Newborn Infant 90. Neonatal Complications of Prematurity 91. Rh Disease and Other Isoimmunization 92. Injuries to the Fetus and Newborn 93. Meconium Aspiration, Cerebral Palsy, and Other Diseases of the Fetus and Newborn 94. Stillbirth Appendix A: Diagnostic Indices in Pregnancy Appendix B: Ultrasound Reference Tables Appendix C: Radiation Dosimetry Appendix D: Umbilical Cord Blood Gas Analysis Index .
Subjects	Pregnancy Complications--Handbooks.
Notes	Rev. ed. of: William's manual of obstetrics / Kenneth J. Leveno ... [et al.]. 22nd ed. c2007. Derived from: Williams obstetrics. 23rd ed. / [edited by] F. Gary Cunningham ... [et al.]. c2010. Includes bibliographical references and index.

Zuzu's petals: a true story of second chances
LCCN	2010936392
Type of material	Book
Personal name	Larsen, Lauren Ward, author.
Main title	Zuzu's petals: a true story of second chances / Lauren Ward Larsen.
Edition	First edition.
Published/Produced	Boulder, Colorado: In the Telling Press, [2011]

	©2011
Description	355 pages; 23 cm
ISBN	9780982990704 (hardback)
LC classification	RG575.5 .L37 2011
Subjects	Larsen, Lauren Ward--Health.
	Pregnancy--Complications.
	Preeclampsia--Patients--Biography.
	Life change events.

RELATED NOVA PUBLICATIONS

CONTROVERSIES IN PREECLAMPSIA

Eyal Sheiner[1] and Yariv Yogev[2]
[1] Residency Program, Soroka University Medical Center, Professor,
Obstetrics and Gynecology, Soroka University Medical Center,
Ben-Gurion University of the Negev, Beer-Sheva, Israel
[2] Rabin Medical Center, Petach Tikva
Sackler Faculty of Medicine, Tel Aviv University, Tel Aviv, Israel

Series: Obstetrics and Gynecology Advances
Publication Date: March 2014   Hardcover ISBN: 978-1-62948-825-7
                                 ebook ISBN: 978-1-62948-828-8

Hypertensive disorders complicate 5-10% of pregnancies and are a leading cause of maternal and perinatal morbidity and mortality. This book serves to highlight the increasing importance of hypertensive disorders in pregnancy across the health care continuum.

It provides a comprehensive, evidenced-based and updated review of controversy aspects relating to preeclampsia and other hypertensive complications in pregnancy. It starts with a broad overview of preeclampsia including an extensive introduction explaining definitions and epidemiology of the disease, and the differential diagnosis of preeclampsia. Risk factors such as obesity and diabetes as well as multifetal gestations are presented in separate chapters. Basic concepts dealing with the pathogenesis of the disease are thoroughly covered including the role of adipokines in preeclampsia. Specific attention is given to prediction and prevention of preeclampsia. The book concludes with short and long term maternal outcome.

Written by international experts, this book is a valuable resource for a broad spectrum of clinicians and healthcare professionals dealing with maternal fetal medicine. Medical and nursing students as well as residents in obstetrics and gynecology, and family practice will also benefit from it at any stage of their training.

THE MOLECULAR DETERMINANTS OF PREECLAMPSIA ACCOUNTABLE FOR MULTIFACTORIAL DISORDER IN PREGNANT WOMEN[*]

Md. Alauddin[1], PhD, and Yearul Kabir[2,†], PhD

[1]Department of Nutrition and Food Technology,
Jashore University of Science and Technology, Jashore, Bangladesh.,
[2]Department of Biochemistry and Molecular Biology,
University of Dhaka, Dhaka, Bangladesh

Multifactorial disorder preeclampsia affects 3-10% of pregnant women worldwide. The main manifestations is oxidative stress, hypertension,

---

[*] The full version of this chapter can be found in *Trends in Biochemistry and Molecular Biology*, edited by Hossain Uddin Shekhar and M. M. Towhidul Islam, published by Nova Science Publishers, Inc, New York, 2019.
[†] Corresponding Author Email: ykabir@yahoo.com.

micoangiopathy, alteration of micro RNA, amino acid, bioactive compound and proteinuria. Preeclampsia is accompanied by the molecular growth restraint within the uterus and premature birth. Moreover opposing confinement consequences who suffered with preeclampsia have an amplified danger of forthcoming health difficulties. Thus this disorder is a foremost reason of maternal and fetal indisposition and their death worldwide. Recent thrilling scientific research have contributed a better molecular understanding of the preclampsia disorder. Epidemiological along with molecular and therapeutic investigation on preeclampsia-based scientific report have provided persuasive suggestion on circulating metabolic factors to preeclampsia disorder. This review paper highlights the role of key molecular factors as well as biomarkers and their mechanism for preeclampsia. This chapter also summarized the recent knowledge of new potential molecular determinants for better understanding of preeclampsia.

RISK FACTORS FOR PREECLAMPSIA IN A HIGH-RISK COHORT OF WOMEN SERVED BY A NURSING-BASED HOME VISITING PROGRAM[*]

Candace Tannis[†], MD, MPH, Rachel Fletcher-Slater, MPH, Inessa Lopez, MPH, Alexandrah Gichingiri, BS, Mario Cassara, MPH, Susanne Lachapelle, RN and Elizabeth Garland, MD, MS

Department of Environmental Medicine and Public Health,
Icahn School of Medicine at Mount Sinai and LSA Family
Health Services, New York, United States of America

In this chapter we aimed to identify the impact of psychosocial risk factors on pregnancy outcomes for high risk women in an urban setting. Women in this category tend to experience adverse pregnancy outcomes, like preeclampsia, at greater rates than low or medium risk women. A retrospective paper chart review of East Harlem women served by LSA Family Health Service (LSA) Maternal Outreach Program (MOP) was conducted. All women who enrolled in the MOP with a singleton pregnancy from January 2015 to December 2017, were eligible for inclusion in our analyses. Data were analyzed using SPSS (version 23). Of 379 total charts reviewed, 68.6% (n=203) were Hispanic/Latina women, 44.8% (n=163) were English only speakers, 67.4% (n=226) were identified as overweight/obese, 90.6% (n=328) were mothers over the age of 20 among those for whom data were available. Sixty-two percent (n=235) initiated prenatal care in their first trimester, and 71.5% (n=271) were

---

[*] The full version of this chapter can be found in *Public Health: Environment and Child Health in a Changing World*, edited by I. Leslie Rubin and Joav Merrick, published by Nova Science Publishers, Inc, New York, 2019.
[†] Correspondence: Candace Tannis MD, MPH, Department of Environmental Medicine and Public Health, Icahn School of Medicine at Mount Sinai, 1 Gustave L Levy Place, New York, NY 10029, United States. Email: Candace.Tannis@mssm.edu.

referred to the MOP by a hospital or other healthcare provider. The percentage of preeclampsia among mothers was 26.9% (n=102). After adjustment for type of LSA services received, and race/ethnicity, there were no associations between psychosocial risk factors and preeclampsia diagnosis in this population. Further research is needed on the relationship between psychosocial risk factors and preeclampsia to identify potential areas of intervention and reduce the burden of disease.

INOSITOLS AND PREECLAMPSIA[*]

Marco Scioscia[†]
Department of Obstetrics and Gynaecology, Policlinico Hospital, Abano Terme, Padua, Italy

Preeclampsia is a disease of human pregnancy charcterized by hypertension and proteinuria. It may have a serious impact on pregnancy outcome, maternal health, and fetal wellbeing. Preeclampsia results from a complex interaction between immunological alterations, endothelial dysfunction, metabolic disturbances, and insulin resistance. Inositol derivates are known to be deeply involved in metabolic signaling and are highly expressed during preeclampsia on both maternal and fetal side. In the past two decades, several studies were published on different aspects where these molecules are involved and these studies demonstrated the relevance of inositols in many aspects of this syndrome. It appears that maternal increase of inositol phosphoglycans P-type in all tissues and fluids reflects an increased production of inositol mediators on the fetal side in preeclampsia that spill over the placenta into the maternal circulation contributing to the onset and mantainace of the syndrome.

---

[*] The full version of this chapter can be found in *Inositols: Guide to Practical Applications in Obstetrics and Gynecology*, edited by Vittorio Unfer, published by Nova Science Publishers, Inc, New York, 2019.
[†] Corresponding author address. E-mail: marcoscioscia@gmail.com.

CARDIOVASCULAR AND RENAL RISKS
AFTER PREECLAMPSIA[*]

Rose Gasnier, MD, MSc
Hospital de Clínicas de Porto alegre,
Universidade Federal do Rio Grande do Sul, Brazil
Wolfson Medical Center,
Sackler University, Tel Aviv, Israel

Population-based studies have shown that women with a history of preeclampsia (PE) have a 2-fold increased risk of long-term cardiovascular disease (CVD). Systematic reviews reported doubled risk of ischemic heart disease (IHD), cerebral vascular accident (CVA) and mortality from CVD after preeclampsia. In addition, women after preeclampsia have 5-12 fold increased risk of developing end-stage renal disease (ESRD) later in life. Recognized guidelines acknowledged preeclampsia as a women-specific risk factor for CVD. Preeclamptic women develop chronic arterial hypertension (CAH) and CVD 6-8 years earlier compared with women with a history of normotensive pregnancy.

Adaptation to pregnancy demands increased cardiovascular and renal effort and it has been proposed that pregnancy is a stress test for the cardiovascular system. The increased cardiovascular and renal risks might be caused by common factor risks that preeclampsia shares with CVD and chronic kidney disease (CKD) as oxidative stress and metabolic alterations. There is a common pathophysiologic pathway of endothelial dysfunction linking placental and vascular disorders. Women with a previous early-onset preeclampsia seem to have a less favorable CVD risk profile, compared to women with late-onset and gestational hypertension, particularly reflected in glucose and lipid levels. Recently papers have found correlation between antiangiogenic protein production and

---

[*] The full version of this chapter can be found in *Horizons in World Cardiovascular Research*. Volume 11, edited by Eleanor H. Bennington, published by Nova Science Publishers, Inc, New York, 2017.

preeclampsia. In this setting, VEGF (vascular endothelial growth factor) is important for the maintenance of glomerular function, and the dysfunction can persist after pregnancy.

During preeclampsia, the kidneys are affected by systemic endothelial dysfunction leading to proteinuria and glomerular endotheliosis, and a lower glomerular filtration rate (GFR) is observed. After termination of pregnancy, the renal disturbances normalize but do not resolve completely in part of the cases. Persistent disturbances in albuminuria and renal function may contribute to the increased risk of cardiovascular and renal disease. Podocyturia may persist postpartum, despite resolution of proteinuria. Viable urinary podocytes have been documented in a variety of glomerular diseases, particularly during the active phases, and plays a major role in the pathogenesis of focal segmental glomerular sclerosis, which is a dominant finding in renal biopsies of women with history of preeclampsia and persistent proteinuria.

Recognition of the hypertensive pregnancy as a risk factor allows identification of a young population of women at risk, with possibility of screening planning and prevention. Besides, understanding the extent and severity of cardiovascular changes has brought new insights into the optimal management of women with preeclampsia: the postpartum recovery from preeclampsia is compromised by asymptomatic cardiovascular dysfunction. Maybe these women need new screening planning with delineation of cardiac functional as predictor of cardiovascular risk in the future.

Related Nova Publications

USE OF ALPHA-FETOPROTEIN FOR DETECTION OF PREECLAMPSIA[*]

Jonathan B. Carmichael[†], PhD and David A. Krantz, MA
PerkinElmer Labs/NTD, Melville, NY, US

Preeclampsia is a leading cause of morbidity and mortality in pregnancy. Alpha-fetoprotein has been used traditionally in the identification of individuals at risk for open neural tube disorders and aneuploidy. Recent evidence suggests that AFP has proangiogenic properties, potentially at the stage of spiral artery invasion. As such, AFP may play an integral role in identification of pregnancies at risk for early onset preeclampsia.

---

[*] The full version of this chapter can be found in *Alpha-fetoprotein: Functions and Clinical Applications*, edited by Nisha Lakhi and Michael Moretti, published by Nova Science Publishers, Inc, New York, 2016.
[†] Corresponding Author address: PekinElmer Labs/NTD, 80 Ruland Road, Suite 1, Melville, N.Y., 11747, US, Email: jon.carmichael@perkinelmer.com.

Prolonged Excitation of Hypothlamic Sympathetic Center Provokes Preeclampsia by the Stimulation of Expanded Pregnant Uterus through Uterus-Brain Nerve[*]

Kazuo Maeda[†]*, MD, PhD*
Department of Obstetrics and Gynecology (Emeritus),
Tottori University Medical School, Yonago, Japan

Two channel electroencephalograph (EEG) machine was made by the author's hand to study EEG of eclampsia and preeclampsia in 1949, when no commercial EEG machine was provided in Japan. As frontal and occipital EEG waves synchronized in eclampsia, and in rabbit's cortex and hypothalamus, It was concluded that excited hypothalamus controlled whole cortex to develop eclamptic attack. As rabbits' hypertension and proteinuria appeared by electric stimulation of sympathetic center of hypothalamus using Kurotsu's electrode, it was noted that preeclampsia appeared when pregnant uterus enlarged to 20 or more gestational weeks and disappeared when the uterus recovered to non-pregnant size after birth, and also enlarged uterus of complete hydatidiform mole developed hypertension and proteinuria without fetus, when the uterus enlarged to the size of 20 weeks' pregnancy, it was speculated that human preeclampsia was caused by excited sympathetic center stimulated by expanded pregnant uterus. However, the route of hypothalamic stimulation was unknown in the study, while fortunately, the presence of the nerve connecting uterus and brain was reorted recently in animal, thus, the author concluded that the preeclampsia is caused by excited hypothalamic sympathetic center, which was stimulated through uterus-brain nerve by expanded pregnant uterus. Sympathetic excitation causes constriction of peripheral arteries

---

[*] The full version of this chapter can be found in *Advances in Medicine and Biology. Volume 109*, edited by Leon V. Berhardt, published by Nova Science Publishers, Inc, New York, 2016.
[†] E-mail: maedak@mocha.ocn.ne.jp, Phone/FAX: 81859-22-6586.

causing hypertension and proteinuria, various metabolic and pathologic changes of preeclampsia, e.g., the constriction of uterine artery reduced maternal uterine arterial blood supply to placenta to develop placental insufficiency, fetal growth restriction (FGR), fetal hypoxia and finally fetal demise. Preeclamptic women will be treated by anti-sympathicotonic drug and sedation of uterus to brain nerve in the future.

STUDIES ON CIRCADIAN PATTERN OF BLOOD PRESSURE IN NORMOTENSIVE PREGNANT WOMEN AND PREECLAMPSIA. IN MEMORY OF LATE PROFESSOR FRANZ HALBERG, FATHER OF CHRONOBIOLOGY*

R. K. Singh[†,1,4], N. S. Verma[2], Neelam Barnwal[3], H. P. Gupta[3], Urmila Singh[3], Seema Mehrotra[3], Ranjana Singh[1] and R. B. Singh[5]

Departments of [1]Biochemistry, [2]Physiology and [3]Obstetrics & Gynecology, King George's Medical University, Lucknow,
[4]Department of Biochemistry, SGRRIM & HS, Dehradun,
[5]Halberg Hospital and Research Institute, Moradabad, India

With the aim of comparing the circadian characteristics of blood pressure (BP) in normotensive pregnant women and preeclampsia, a total of 35 pregnant women with gestational age more than 20 weeks (age: 18-40 years) were recruited from the patients admitted in the Department of

---

* The full version of this chapter can be found in *Chronocardiology and Cardiac Research*, edited by Krasimira Hristova, Jan Fedacko, Germaine Cornelissen, and Ram B. Singh, published by Nova Science Publishers, Inc, New York, 2016.
† Address for correspondence: Dr R K Singh, Professor and Head, Biochemistry Department, Shri Guru Ram Rai Institute of Medical & Health Sciences, Dehradun – 248001 (Uttarakhand), INDIA. Phone: +91-135-2522168 O); Fax: +91-135-2522117 Email singhrk23a@hotmail.com

Obstetrics & Gynecology, Queen Mary's Hospital, King George's Medical University, Lucknow. In these patients, systolic (S) BP was 140 mmHg or above and diastolic (D) BP was 90 mmHg or above on 2 consecutive occasions, with measurements taken 6 hours apart. Thirty five age-matched pregnant women were diagnosed as 'normotensive', when their casual BP was always below 140/90 mmHg on at least 3 different occasions were included as Controls. We analyzed BP records obtained by ABPM (TM-2430 monitors from the A&D Company, Tokyo, Japan) for 3 days, observing all the required precautions and after getting their informed consent and proper counseling. Compared with normotensive pregnancies, a statistically significant elevation of the circadian rhythm-adjusted mean (MESOR, a rhythm-adjusted average value) of BP was observed in preeclampsia ($p < 0.001$ for both SBP and DBP).

THE PATHOGENESIS OF HELLP SYNDROME: SIMILARITIES AND DIFFERENCES WITH PREECLAMPSIA[*]

Babbette LaMarca[†]

Maternal Fetal Medicine Fellowship Program,
The University of Mississippi Medical Center
Jackson, MS, USA

Even though HELLP syndrome is considered a distinct type of preeclampsia that has been known to us for more than three decades, there is much that remains unknown about its pathogenesis and pathophysiology. What is known will be summarized in the following review with the intention of delineating the differences between preeclampsia and HELLP

---

[*] The full version of this chapter can be found in *The 2015 Compendium for HELLP Syndrome: From Bench to Bedside*, edited by James N. Martin, Jr., published by Nova Science Publishers, Inc, New York, 2015.
[†] Corresponding author: bblamarca@umc.edu.

syndrome. Many studies have been performed during the last decade to address the gaps in our knowledge. There are a number of promising new directions that research will take us over the coming years to more fully clarify the important features of HELLP syndrome, a disorder which greatly impacts maternal and perinatal morbidity and mortality on a global scale.

HYPERTENSION AND PREECLAMPSIA[*]

Laura Baños Cándenas[1], Pedro Azumendi Gómez[2] and Daniel Abehsera Davó[1,]*

[1]Obstetrics and Gynecology Department. Quirón University Hospital. Málaga. Spain
[2]Obstetrics and Gynecology Department. Regional University Hospital of Málaga. Málaga. Spain

Hypertensive disorders of pregnancy are an important cause of severe morbidity, long-term disability and death among both mothers and their babies. Among the hypertensive disorders that complicate pregnancy, pre-eclampsia and eclampsia stand out as major causes of maternal and perinatal mortality and morbidity. Hypertensive disorders during pregnancy occur in women with pre-existing primary or secondary chronic hypertension, and in women who develop new-onset hypertension in the second half of pregnancy. Hypertensive disorders during pregnancy carry risks for the woman and the baby.. Women with early-onset pre-eclampsia require admission to a tertiary care facility for treatment and one-third experience complications that may necessitate intensive care. Infants are often delivered preterm, need prolonged intensive care and develop

---

[*] The full version of this chapter can be found in *Handbook for High Risk Pregnancy: Clinical Management*, edited by Ernesto González-Mesa and Daniel Abehsera., published by Nova Science Publishers, Inc, New York, 2015.
[*] Corresponding author: Email: laurabc84@hotmail.es.

complications, including lifelong disability, giving rise to large healthcare costs. Early identification of women at risk is a key aim of antenatal care.

INDEX

A

abuse, 136
accommodations, 128
acute mountain sickness, 105
adaptation, 24, 56, 84, 105, 137
adaptations, 134
adhesion, 22, 23, 26
adjustment, 140, 169
advancement, 39
adverse conditions, 62
age, 14, 60, 61, 62, 63, 70, 104, 107, 121, 130, 135, 151, 154, 158, 168, 174
aggregation, 33
albuminuria, 171
alkaline phosphatase, 58
American Heart Association, 73, 75
amino acid, 167
amniocentesis, 124, 127
amniotic fluid, 83, 96, 118, 121, 127
amplitude, 8, 41
anesthetics, 128
aneuploidy, 172
aneurysm, 96, 146
angiogenesis, 27
angiotensin converting enzyme, 30
angiotensin II, 30
animal modeling, vii, viii, 19, 20
anticoagulation, 147
anticonvulsant, 66
antihypertensive drugs, 25, 38, 41, 48, 49, 51, 60, 62, 64, 65, 68, 69
antioxidant, 26, 29, 34, 159
anxiety, 143, 144
anxiety disorder, 143, 144
aortic stenosis, 146
apoptosis, 23, 28, 29
arrhythmia, 46
arterial hypertension, ix, 5, 6, 13, 53, 58, 65, 75, 170
arteries, 21, 22, 24, 32, 40, 49, 56, 173
arteriosclerosis, 80, 81
arteriovenous malformation, 95
artery, 2, 24, 29, 32, 147, 172, 174
aspiration, 95, 146
assessment, 42, 58, 59, 109, 120, 134, 145
asthma, 148
asymptomatic, 171
atherosclerosis, 9, 30, 105
atrial fibrillation, 95, 114
attachment, 137

autoantibodies, 30, 91
autoimmune disease, 23
autonomic nervous regulation, 38, 42, 46, 47, 48
autonomic nervous system, 38, 39, 47

B

bacterial infection, 142
baroreceptor, 92
behavioral problems, 105
beneficial effect, 26
benefits, 59, 64, 130, 151
beta-carotene, 26
bilirubin, 58
biomarkers, 7, 12, 32, 52, 167
birth control, 125
bleeding, 55, 101, 103, 112, 126, 138, 149
blood, viii, 1, 3, 7, 11, 21, 22, 25, 26, 28, 29, 40, 42, 44, 46, 47, 49, 55, 56, 57, 58, 59, 60, 62, 63, 64, 65, 68, 80, 82, 93, 118, 127, 152, 174
blood flow, 21, 22, 26, 29, 44, 46, 58, 60, 64
blood pressure, viii, 1, 25, 40, 49, 55, 56, 57, 58, 60, 62, 63, 64, 65, 68, 80, 82, 93, 174
body mass index, viii, 1, 4, 26
Body mass index, 4, 5, 6, 7, 13
Body Mass Index (BMI), 4, 5, 6, 7, 13
body weight, 10, 125
brain, 57, 59, 146, 173
breastfeeding, 124, 127, 140
breathing, 42, 83, 127

C

caesarean section, 6
calcium channel blocker, 65
capillary, 26, 30
carbohydrates, 134

carcinogenesis, 158
cardiovascular disease, ix, 35, 38, 52, 54, 68, 69, 80, 113, 115, 154, 159, 170
cardiovascular risk, 98, 113, 155, 171
cardiovascular system, 49, 170
catabolism, 157
central maternal hemodynamics, ix, 37, 38, 41
central nervous system, 28
centralisation, 45
cerebral hemorrhage, 68
cervical dysplasia, 101, 103
cervix, 60, 61, 62, 63, 126
cesarean section, 60, 62, 63, 96, 111, 124
chemical, 26, 111
childhood sexual abuse, 137
children, 131, 152, 155
Chi-square Automatic Interaction Detection (CHAID), 12
cholestasis, 141
chromosome, 8, 25, 108
chronic diseases, 105
chronic kidney disease (CKD), 170
chronic venous insufficiency, 38
circulation, ix, 23, 27, 28, 30, 37, 38, 39, 46, 49, 64, 84, 94, 169
CKD, 92
clarity, 67
classes, 4, 22, 127
classification, 12, 79, 82, 85, 87, 89, 91, 94, 98, 100, 102, 104, 106, 108, 109, 111, 113, 114, 116, 119, 120, 121, 122, 123, 124, 133, 143, 145, 148, 149, 150, 154, 156, 157, 164
clinical problems, 83
coagulation profile, 42
color, 82, 89, 91, 115, 116, 160
commercial, 173
communication, 22, 84, 112, 117

Index

complications, ix, 7, 15, 39, 40, 54, 61, 64, 81, 89, 93, 101, 103, 120, 138, 154, 159, 160, 166, 176
compounds, 41
compression, 43
conception, 77
conference, 159
confinement, 167
conflict of interest, 62
congestive heart failure, 105
consensus, 67, 69, 70
contraceptives, 105, 149
control group, 4, 5, 6, 9, 10, 11, 12, 25
controversies, 87, 90
coronary heart disease, 113
correlation, 4, 5, 6, 10, 12, 44, 46, 170
correlation analysis, 4, 12
corticosteroids, ix, 54, 61, 68, 69
counseling, 135, 151, 175
craniotomy, 96, 145
creatinine, 40, 58
cross-sectional study, 51
cytochrome, 157
cytokines, 22, 23, 24, 28, 38, 46, 47, 49

D

danger, 167
data analysis, 4
DBP, 55, 65, 175
deaths, 38, 66, 72, 73, 157
defects, 84, 107, 109, 152
delivery, viii, ix, 1, 2, 6, 7, 13, 14, 38, 48, 50, 53, 54, 55, 56, 62, 63, 69, 71, 73, 77, 96, 107, 109, 111, 120, 121, 124, 153, 160, 161
depression, 98, 140, 148, 153, 155
depth, 92, 94, 95, 101, 103
detection, 24, 39, 58, 118
diabetes, 22, 40, 98, 100, 101, 103, 126, 139, 146, 148, 149, 152, 154, 159, 166

diagnostic criteria, 69
diaphragmatic hernia, 146
diastolic blood pressure, 10, 55, 58, 59, 64
diastolic pressure, 62
diet, 25, 104, 126, 158
differential diagnosis, ix, 53, 58, 166
Disintegrin and metalloproteinase domain-containing protein 12 (ADAM12), 4, 7, 8, 9, 12, 13
diseases, 27, 33, 40, 49, 80, 81, 96, 101, 103, 106, 110, 112, 114, 142, 171
Disintegrin and metalloproteinase domain-containing protein 12, 4, 7, 8, 9, 12, 13
disorder, 20, 32, 50, 143, 149, 166, 176
disseminated intravascular coagulation, 95
domestic violence, 140
dominance, 42
doppler, 32, 60
Down syndrome, 8, 130
drug treatment, 65
drugs, 39, 48, 51, 65, 101, 103, 125, 136, 151
dyslipidemia, 47

E

early labor, 138
early predictors, 2, 3, 12
Eastern Europe, 77
economic development, 38
ectopic pregnancy, 101, 103, 150
edema, 30, 59, 61, 94
editors, 82, 91, 113, 115, 160
education, 115, 137
electrolyte imbalance, 47
embolus, 96, 132
emergency, 60, 111, 114, 149
endocrinology, 101, 103
endothelial cells, 27, 28
endothelial dysfunction, 22, 24, 26, 27, 29, 30, 47, 56, 169, 170, 171

endothelium, 26, 27, 30, 34, 47
end-stage renal disease, 170
enzyme immunoassay, 3
epidemic, 98, 104
epidemiologic, 106
epidemiology, 99, 107, 113, 166
epidural hematoma, 96
erythroblastosis fetalis, 121
estrogen, 113
etiology, ix, 53, 87, 90, 93, 106, 122
evacuation, 96
evidence, ix, 53, 67, 100, 102, 160, 172
evolution, 84, 104, 106
exclusion, 40
exercise, 83, 125, 140, 158
exposure, 23, 56, 156
extracellular matrix, 22

F

families, 33, 151
fertility, 99, 107, 140, 151
fertilization, 151, 155
fetal abnormalities, 132
fetal distress, ix, 37, 38, 45, 46, 47, 48, 51, 83
fetal growth, 8, 14, 21, 48, 58, 64, 65, 107, 131, 138, 174
fetus, ix, 3, 20, 27, 39, 46, 48, 53, 56, 57, 59, 60, 61, 62, 64, 74, 84, 109, 134, 173
fluid, 45, 47, 127, 138, 145
food, 124, 126, 134
foundations, 133

G

gastroenteritis, 132
gene expression, 158
gene therapy, 83
general anesthesia, 96

genes, 24, 25, 33, 117
genetic factors, 21, 33
genetic predisposition, 26
genetic screening, 124, 135
genetics, 106, 107, 108
gestation, viii, 1, 2, 3, 4, 6, 12, 13, 21, 45, 49, 57, 58, 62, 63, 64, 68, 70, 72, 74, 84, 139, 149
gestational age, 11, 39, 60, 61, 62, 63, 64, 68, 69, 134, 174
gestational diabetes, 83, 99, 139
global scale, 176
globalization, 98
growth, ix, 9, 14, 16, 25, 26, 27, 32, 34, 35, 42, 43, 45, 48, 53, 56, 59, 71, 73, 84, 121, 126, 138, 149, 155, 167
growth factor, ix, 9, 14, 16, 25, 26, 27, 35, 53, 56, 71, 73
growth hormone, 84
guidelines, 55, 65, 67, 70, 104, 160, 170
gynecologist, 75, 76, 78

H

hair, 129
hair loss, 130
hay fever, 131
hazards, 125
health, 52, 60, 62, 68, 81, 83, 98, 103, 104, 107, 124, 125, 134, 144, 150, 151, 154, 155, 157, 165, 167, 169
health care, 144, 152, 165
health education, 137
health problems, 141
health risks, 150
heart attack, 80
heart disease, 108, 113, 170
heart failure, 148
heart rate, vii, viii, ix, 37, 38, 39, 51, 62, 113, 129

Index

heart rate variability, vii, viii, ix, 37, 38, 39, 51
hellp syndrome, 50
hematocrit, 59, 61
hemoglobinopathies, 160
hemophilia a, 95
hemorrhage, 49, 94, 120, 138, 149
hemostasis, 23, 26, 47, 109
hepatitis, 77
high blood pressure, 54, 56, 64, 68, 79
High Risk Pregnancy, 176
history, viii, 2, 13, 68, 69, 87, 90, 106, 125, 134, 170, 171
home visiting, 168
HPV, 76, 101, 103
human, vii, viii, 4, 16, 17, 19, 20, 27, 40, 49, 83, 105, 106, 107, 117, 140, 158, 169, 173
human body, 105
human chorionic gonadotropin, 4
hydatidiform mole, 173
Hydrargyrum (HG), 13, 139
hydrops, 23
hyperemesis, 139
hypertension, viii, ix, 2, 5, 6, 13, 14, 19, 20, 22, 25, 32, 34, 35, 40, 50, 53, 54, 55, 56, 57, 58, 59, 61, 64, 65, 67, 68, 69, 70, 72, 73, 74, 75, 77, 79, 80, 81, 82, 85, 87, 89, 90, 91, 92, 93, 101, 103, 110, 114, 115, 116, 120, 132, 139, 148, 149, 157, 160, 161, 166, 169, 170, 173, 176
hyperthyroidism, 142
hypothesis, 20, 23, 28, 32
hypoxia, 27, 28, 29, 56, 64, 83, 174

I

ideal, 125
identification, 92, 171, 172
ileostomy, 148
image, 133, 137
imaging modalities, 112
imbalances, 29
immune response, 14, 24
immunodeficiency, 112, 132
imprinting, 99
In vitro fertilisation (IVF), 11, 151
in vivo, 28, 158
induction, 60, 61, 62, 63, 128, 153
inertia, 105
infant care, 105
infant mortality, viii, 19, 20, 107
infants, 14, 84
infarction, 23
infection, 48, 76, 77, 109, 131, 141, 148, 149, 159
infertility, 101, 103
inflammation, 11, 26, 28, 29, 34, 35, 47, 51
inflammatory disease, 28, 150
inflammatory mediators, 47
informed consent, 40, 175
injections, 68
injury, 23, 29, 95, 146
inositol, 169
insulin, 9, 169
insulin resistance, 169
intensive care unit, 61, 62, 129
interface, 117
interferon, 33
intervention, 48, 49, 62, 92, 136, 169
intimacy, 152
intracellular calcium, 24
intracerebral hemorrhage, 65
intrauterine growth retardation (IUGR), 2, 32
intravenous fluids, 68
ischemia, 22, 23, 29, 39, 56
issues, 50, 120, 124, 134
Italy, 169

J

jaundice, 48
Jordan, 133, 134

K

ketoacidosis, 96, 148
kidney, 5, 22, 28, 57, 70, 85, 86, 88, 91, 92, 93, 96, 131
kidney transplantation, 96

L

laboratory tests, 60
lactation, 130, 140
laparoscopic surgery, 95
latency, 158
lead, 12, 29
learning, 94
leukocytes, 23, 28
lifestyle changes, 80, 81, 125
ligament, 132, 136
lipid metabolism, 11, 47
lipid peroxidation, 26, 29, 34, 42, 47
lipids, 9, 16, 30, 42, 50
liver, 28, 40, 57, 58, 59, 62, 76, 77, 88, 91
liver enzymes, 62
local anesthetic, 97
low platelet count, 47
low-density lipoprotein, 35
lupus erythematosus, 149

M

macrophages, 28, 30
magnesium, ix, 25, 47, 54, 60, 61, 62, 64, 66, 67, 68, 69, 71
magnesium sulphate, ix, 54, 66, 67, 71
magnet, 132
magnitude, 80
majority, 44
management, vii, viii, ix, 13, 37, 39, 49, 52, 53, 60, 61, 63, 65, 67, 72, 74, 75, 80, 91, 92, 95, 99, 100, 102, 112, 135, 145, 147, 160, 171
mapping, 144
mass, 4, 22, 94, 112, 146, 149
matrix, 22
mean arterial pressure, 13
measurement, 8, 58, 60
mechanical ventilation, 68
medical, 2, 15, 22, 40, 61, 80, 96, 123, 152, 154
medical care, 152
medicine, 39, 67, 85, 94, 100, 102, 103, 104, 116, 146, 156, 166
Medium arterial pressure (MAP), 5, 6, 7, 13
mellitus, 22, 40, 98, 101, 103, 148, 154
membranes, 23, 149
Metabolic, 20, 25, 88, 90, 93, 134
metabolic disturbances, 169
metabolic syndrome, 40
metabolism, 9, 47, 99, 158
metalloproteinase, viii, 1, 4
methamphetamine, 95
methodology, 40, 100, 102
micronutrients, 40, 42, 47
miscommunication, 135
mitochondria, 84
mitral stenosis, 96
models, 13, 88, 90
modern science, ix, 53
molecular biology, 33
molecules, 22, 29, 169
morbidity, 2, 12, 38, 55, 93, 107, 140, 155, 165, 172, 176
mortality, 2, 38, 55, 61, 65, 69, 74, 75, 93, 107, 140, 165, 170, 172, 176
mRNA, 23, 30
multiple sclerosis, 142

Index

N

natural killer (NK) cells, 24
nausea, 151
necrosis, 23, 27, 28
negative consequences, 3
nervous system, 158
neurodegenerative disorders, 159
neurophysiology, 120
neutrophils, 23
New Zealand, 64, 67, 72, 74
next generation, 118
nitric oxide, 26, 34, 158
nitrite, 26
NK cells, 24
non-classical, 24
nurses, 101, 103
nursing, 143, 147, 166
nutrition, 27, 104, 134, 151
nutritional assessment, 134

O

obesity, 25, 98, 105, 118, 142, 166
operations, 96
organ, ix, 37, 38, 44, 56, 57, 59, 65, 158
outpatient, 61, 94, 97
ovarian cancer, 101, 103
overweight, 4, 15, 168
ovulation, 125, 140
oxidative stress, 26, 28, 29, 30, 32, 34, 35, 38, 47, 52, 83, 88, 158, 166, 170

P

pain, 94, 97, 101, 103, 111, 126, 135, 148, 149
palm oil, 158
palpitations, 136
PAPP-A (pregnancy-associated plasma protein A), 4, 14, 49
parallel, 118
parasitic infection, 143
parenthood, 151
parenting, 153
participants, 40
pathogenesis, 1, iii, v, vii, viii, ix, 11, 19, 20, 25, 26, 27, 29, 31, 32, 34, 48, 53, 56, 166, 171, 175
pathology, ix, 5, 35, 110
pathophysiological, 54, 57, 90
pathophysiology, vii, viii, 2, 19, 20, 32, 33, 90, 113, 175
pathway, 51, 157, 170
perinatal, 2, 15, 38, 39, 48, 49, 61, 63, 117, 136, 165, 176
perineum, 128, 140
permeability, 27, 30, 44
pharmaceutical, ix, 37, 39, 48, 49, 136
pharmacological agents, 40
Philadelphia, 111, 115
physical health, 124
physiology, 82, 83, 84, 85, 88, 121, 133, 143, 159
physiopathology, 84, 89, 99
placenta, 9, 16, 17, 20, 23, 27, 28, 29, 30, 31, 32, 35, 57, 59, 87, 90, 96, 117, 121, 128, 134, 152, 161, 169, 174
placenta previa, 96
placental abruption, 58, 61, 64
placental barrier, ix, 37, 39
platelet aggregation, 42, 47
platelet count, 59
platelets, 61, 62
population, 4, 33, 43, 44, 54, 74, 169, 171
postpartum depression, 130
precocious puberty, 101, 103
preeclampsia (PE), v, vii, viii, ix, 1, 2, 3, 4, 5, 6, 7, 8, 9, 10, 11, 12, 13, 14, 15, 16, 17, 19, 20, 21, 22, 23, 24, 25, 26, 27, 28,

29, 30, 31, 32, 33, 34, 35, 38, 39, 40, 42, 43, 44, 45, 46, 47, 48, 49, 50, 51, 52, 53, 54, 55, 56, 57, 58, 59, 60, 62, 63, 64, 66, 68, 69, 70, 71, 73, 74, 75, 77, 80, 81, 83, 86, 87, 90, 93, 95, 99, 101, 103, 105, 107, 108, 110, 111, 113, 115, 116, 118, 119, 120, 121, 122, 123, 127, 139, 144, 147, 148, 149, 152, 154, 157, 159, 161, 164, 165, 166, 168, 169, 170, 171, 172, 173, 174, 175, 176
pregnancy, ix, 2, 3, 4, 5, 6, 7, 8, 10, 12, 13, 14, 15, 16, 17, 20, 21, 23, 24, 26, 27, 28, 29, 30, 33, 34, 35, 38, 39, 42, 45, 46, 47, 49, 50, 54, 55, 56, 57, 58, 60, 61, 62, 63, 64, 67, 68, 69, 70, 72, 73, 74, 77, 83, 87, 89, 90, 91, 99, 101, 103, 106, 107, 108, 109, 111, 114, 115, 116, 117, 120, 121, 122, 123, 124, 125, 134, 149, 150, 151, 154, 156, 157, 159, 160, 165, 166, 168, 169, 170, 171, 172, 173, 176
prematurity, 138, 156
premenstrual syndrome, 105
preservation, 60, 152
preterm delivery, ix, 38, 50, 69, 107, 109
preterm infants, 73
prevention, viii, ix, 3, 19, 39, 40, 48, 49, 51, 54, 61, 67, 68, 69, 97, 113, 139, 159, 166, 171
principles, 67, 135
problem solving, 108
professional literature, 6
professionals, 166
programming, 83, 98, 118
pro-inflammatory, 24, 29, 47, 50
proteins, 28, 30, 42
proteinuria, viii, 10, 19, 20, 30, 40, 54, 55, 56, 58, 60, 167, 169, 171, 173
psychosocial stress, 104
pulmonary contusion, 95
pulmonary edema, 40, 59, 65
pyelonephritis, viii, 2, 5, 6, 13, 141

Q

QT interval, 46
quartile, 4
Queensland, 67

R

race, 169
radicals, 29
random numbers, 3
reactions, 42, 96, 157
reactivity, 27, 29, 31, 42
receptor, 25, 27, 29, 30, 35, 56
recognition, 116
recommendations, iv, 6, 13, 65, 67, 68, 69, 115
recovery, 124, 171
recreational, 125, 137
recurrence, 66
regions of the world, 38
Registry, 69
rehabilitation, 49, 113
rejection, 24
relevance, 169
relief, 120, 153
remission, 20
renal failure, 59, 93, 148
renin, 30, 91
repair, 94, 146
reproduction, 84, 104, 106, 107, 117
requirements, 110, 143
resistance, 9, 21, 27, 38, 39, 41, 98
resolution, 171
respiratory distress syndrome, 68, 69
response, 9, 21, 24, 26, 35, 38, 43, 44, 51, 61
response syndrome, 38
retina, 59
retinol, viii, 1, 4, 16

Index

retinol binding protein 4 (RBP4), 4, 7, 8, 9, 10, 12, 13
rhythm, 58, 60, 175
risk, 5, 6, 7, 10, 12, 13, 14, 15, 16, 22, 25, 26, 38, 42, 48, 49, 52, 61, 62, 63, 64, 65, 66, 68, 69, 81, 101, 103, 107, 113, 135, 155, 168, 170, 171, 172, 177
risk assessment, 52, 135
risk profile, 170
risks, 15, 151, 152, 170, 176

S

safety, 67, 121, 134
salmon, 132
savings, 152
savings account, 152
science, 83, 115, 144
secretion, 24
sensitivity, 12, 13, 26, 30, 42
serum, viii, 1, 3, 10, 14, 15, 16, 17, 40, 42, 49, 73
sexual activity, 84
sexual dimorphism, 84
shape, 22, 92, 126
signs, 5, 23, 26, 28, 45, 56, 57, 59, 61, 62, 69, 125, 140
sinus arrhythmia, ix, 37, 42, 45, 46, 51
sleep apnea, 95
sleep deprivation, 153
smoking cessation, 155
smooth muscle, 21, 26
social relationships, 105
sperm, 116, 125
spine, 121, 133
stability, 27
standard deviation, 41
statistics, 80
stenosis, 23, 146
stimulation, 173
stock, 126
storage, 21
stress, 23, 29, 30, 32, 35, 41, 47, 52, 105, 125, 152, 159, 170
stress response, 23
structure, 21, 29, 55, 133
style, 126
subgroups, 5, 12, 40, 48
substance abuse, 136
substance use, 136
substance use disorders, 137
sulfate, 60, 61, 62, 64, 67, 68, 69
supplementation, 34, 157
suppression, 23, 45, 47
susceptibility, 26, 30, 33, 105
swelling, 129
symptoms, 54, 57, 61
syndrome, 20, 28, 38, 52, 56, 57, 83, 88, 90, 93, 95, 98, 115, 127, 136, 146, 149, 154, 169, 175
systemic inflammatory, 28, 38
systemic lupus erythematosus, 22
systolic blood pressure, 55, 59

T

T cell, 24
tactics, 3, 61
target, 38, 50, 64, 83
target population, 50
Task Force, 55, 74, 75, 114
testing, 43, 71, 108, 109, 127, 135, 151, 152
thalassemia, 108
therapeutic use, 159
therapy, 49, 51, 60, 61, 64, 68, 69, 83, 92, 99, 112, 122, 137
threatened abortion, 6, 7
thrombocytopenia, 30, 40, 59
thrombosis, 23, 132
thyroid, 101, 103, 108, 142
thyroiditis, 142
thyrotoxicosis, 40

tissue, 23, 26, 33
tobacco smoking, 41
tocopherols, 158
total energy, 134
tracheostomy, 95
trainees, 94, 100, 102, 145
training, 101, 103, 166
transaminases, 40, 61
transforming growth factor, 27
treatment, viii, ix, 19, 39, 48, 50, 53, 57, 58, 60, 62, 63, 64, 65, 67, 68, 69, 73, 80, 81, 89, 91, 92, 112, 137, 155, 159, 160, 176
trial, 71, 159
trisomy, 25
tumor progression, 16
twins, 130
tyrosine, ix, 25, 28, 35, 53, 56, 73

U

ulcerative colitis, 148
ultrasonography, 41, 62, 121
ultrasound, 41, 59, 99, 120, 121, 127
United Kingdom, 66, 72, 115
United States, 54, 70, 80, 85, 168
urinary tract, 141
urinary tract infection, 141
uterus, 21, 43, 56, 64, 167, 173

V

vaccinations, 125
vaginitis, 142
variables, ix, 37, 42, 46, 47, 48, 49
variations, 31, 107
vascular diseases, 93
vascular endothelial growth factor (VEGF), 56

vascular system, 9
vasoconstriction, 30, 49, 56, 57
vasodilation, 45
vasopressor, 21
vasospasm, 26
vein, 26, 43, 46, 132
ventilation, 95, 147
vessels, 21, 43
viral infection, 143
vitamin B1, 156
vitamin C, 26
Vitamin C, 26
vitamin E, 26, 157
vitamins, 26, 40, 130
vomiting, 136, 149
vulva, 136

W

water, 128
web, 153
web sites, 153
weight changes, 129
weight gain, 125
well-being, 61, 124, 135
World Health Organization, 67, 75

Z

zinc, 25, 47

ß

ß-subunit human chorionic gonadotropin (ß-HCG), 8